Healing Through
REIKI

DR. BEENA RANI GOEL

ASHWITA GOEL

Health Care Trust
264, Shivabasava Nagar,
Belgaum – 590010, India

Printing History:

4th Edition, 2016
3rd Edition, 2011
2nd Edition, 2007
1st Edition, 2000

Cover Design and Editing:
Ashwita Goel

Dedicated to our family

CONTENTS

ACKNOWLEDGEMENTS

I am eternally indebted to my mother Smt. C.L Rohinikutty and father Sri D. Gopinathan for having given me this body, through which I can strive to attain salvation. My mother's role in providing me with a memorable childhood was pivotal in shaping my life and destiny.

An important milestone in my journey to the philosophical path was initiation to SKY (Simplified Kundalini Yoga) in 1980 by Prof Nagaraj at Manipal. Though I have lost contact with him, let me take this opportunity to record my heartfelt indebtedness to him.

Words are not adequate to express my gratitude to my revered Reiki Teacher Ms. Padma Khetan (Jaipur) who initiated me into the path of Reiki. The example of her life and the peace she exudes are strong inspirations for me. I am also grateful to my friend Minal for being instrumental in my development as a Reiki healer and teacher.

Each and every person whom I have come in contact with has added to my development and improved my understanding of life.

I have learned a lot of lessons, spiritual and otherwise, from my husband and children. Their full-hearted cooperation, understanding and support are the basis for my ventures.

I am grateful to the Almighty for giving me the opportunities and the will to tread the path towards eternal bliss.

Dr. Beena Rani Goel

FOREWORD

It was in April of 1999 on a flight from Chicago to Amsterdam when I randomly sat next to a friendly couple. After a few hours of conversation, we exchanged contact details and parted ways, but unbeknownst to me – thus began my Reiki journey.

Upon my return to England, I received an email from Beena. This was no ordinary correspondence, as she had tapped into some insightful personal characteristics and questions. When I asked her how she knew, she said it was due to Reiki. I was intrigued and tried to gain a deeper understanding of this mysterious concept that seems to make so many people happy. As our communication grew more frequent, the presence of Reiki also increased.

The turning point for me was in June of 2000 when I met Beena in London and she once again showed me the power of Reiki through its energy and insights. Our relationship soon turned into a trusting and loving friendship. I learned so much over time and I was attuned to level I in May 2003. Life has not been the same ever since. The Reiki energy soon began to make its way into my life through the destined channels.

In my experience, Reiki attunements are very different at every level and each one brings greater understanding of the self and the universe we live in. It is a personal journey to inner peace and spiritual development with newfound optimism, but above of all – it is in our own hands. The more one is sincerely open to Reiki, the more endless the possibilities. And if you are truly blessed (as I was), you will meet a soul mate along the way.

Nupur Saxena

PREFACE

Reiki is a powerful, yet the simplest medium to face life with a smile on your face and peace in your heart. With Reiki, one learns to take the responsibility of one's own life and actions. With the level of understanding that Reiki provides, one can see through the suffering and realize how much one's circumstances have been the result of his/her own attitude and deeds.

We ventured into Reiki almost two decades back as a means to deal with simple physical ailments. Gradually we were drawn into it, becoming masters. Having got the opportunity to facilitate healings and attunements to thousands of people across the globe, we are amazed at the ways in which Reiki can work.

Long term physical ailments which showed no improvements despite a vast array of treatments have vanished after 21 days of healing or sometimes much less. We have watched in joy as Reiki healing helped people leave behind suicidal tendencies, improve relationships and bring self-confidence to many youngsters in facing life's challenges.

The best thing we like about Reiki is that it brings to you whatever is needed to improve one's worldly life or spiritual life. Of course it is up to you to take it forward or leave it, because Reiki never forces anything on us, including progress – it has to be sought first. The moment you decide to tread a particular path, Reiki will start helping you in that direction. This is a very powerful aspect of Reiki.

Practicing Reiki is the simplest thing one can imagine. There is absolutely no prerequisites or conditions associated with this non-invasive healing technique. With Western medicine continuing to explore alternative methods of healing, Reiki is becoming popular as a reliable technique and is now being used in several hospitals all over the world. When it is so simple and can improve life beyond expectation, learning Reiki and practicing it daily can help you to enjoy life to the fullest!

This edition has a few changes in the style of healing oneself. Over the years, we have found that the average energy contained in the lower chakras has drastically diminished, possibly due to over-stimulation and fast-paced lifestyles. Consequently, we find that healing from the base chakra and moving upwards helps bring greater balance and stability, and hence this change.

Dr. Beena Rani & Ashwita Goel

August 2016

INTRODUCTION

Being a dentist by profession, it is easy for me to understand that when I render treatment to a patient, the healing is brought about by the energy from the patient's own body. What else could describe all those cases where large areas of bone destruction have healed by new bone formation once I finished treating the affected tooth?

Everything in nature has a capacity to heal itself. If by some means, this self-healing capacity can be geared into full force, there will be hundreds of situations in which we can avoid swallowing tablets.

I have nothing against allopathic medicines. In fact, I use them in my dental practice. They are of tremendous help in crisis situations. However, their overuse can bring us to a blind end, like the one we are currently witnessing with antibiotics. There are so many antibiotic resistant bacteria today, that we are fast approaching the pre-antibiotic era.

I first heard of Reiki while watching a documentary on alternative therapies,. Its philosophy and simplicity appealed to me and I decided to learn it. Then followed months of searching for a teacher. When I finally got the attunement from Ms. Padma Khetan (Jaipur), I felt that the experience during attunement was less than my expectations.

But after a period of regular practice, in retrospection, I was astonished at the changes in me. I realised that apart from being healthier, I was gradually evolving into a better human being as well. I am no longer the introvert that I used to be.

This transformation brought me in contact with people who were suffering and by then, I knew that Reiki could help them. It did. When those who benefited wanted to be Reiki channels, I thought of becoming a Reiki teacher.

Reiki is thus not just for physical healing, but for facilitating shifts in our mental make- up, emotional maturity and spiritual awareness. If we want to change our lives, we must first transform ourselves. And Reiki is the simplest and most powerful means to bring about this inner change.

HISTORY OF REIKI

The information we have about Reiki is constantly changing. Reiki masters like Frank Arjava Petter, William L. Rand, Frans Stein and many others have done a lot of work in this area to give more complete and factual information about Reiki. New information and facts about Reiki in Japan has also added to the understanding of Reiki's history.

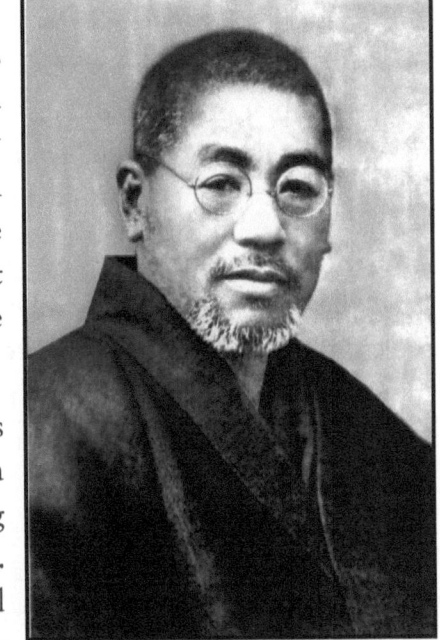

It was believed for many years that the practice of Reiki had died out in Japan but now new information about Reiki in Japan is coming to light. The Japanese Reiki system is slightly different from the Reiki that is used in the west.

What we do know for a fact is that Reiki was "rediscovered" in Japan by Dr Mikao Usui during the beginning of the 20th century. The three persons who play a vital role in the history of Reiki are Dr Mikao Usui, Dr Hayashi, and Mrs Hawayo Takata.

Mikao Usui

Mikao Usui was born into a family with the Samurai legacy (Hatamoto). At age 4 he began his studies at a monastery of Tendai Buddhism. By 1877, he was very accomplished in martial arts. He married at age 30 and had a son and daughter.

Mikao Usui travelled extensively and studied many concepts before discovering Reiki. He took what he studied and combined what seemed right into the Usui system of healing. When his life was not going well, he decided to go to Mt. Kurama to meditate for answers. Perhaps he was looking for a personal transformation for which the mountain was noted and for help in healing his life. He opened himself to the higher power and not only received healing for himself, but a way to help others too.

He chose a place near a watercourse on Mount Kurama in Japan and kept twenty-one small stones near him to mark the time. At the end of each day he would throw away one stone. On the twenty-first day just before dawn, Usui saw a projectile of light coming towards him at great speed. His first impulse was to run away but on second thoughts, he decided to accept what was coming as answer to his meditation, even if it resulted in death.

The light struck his third eye and he lost consciousness for a time. Then he saw millions of rainbow bubbles and finally, as if on a screen, the Reiki symbols appeared in golden letters and he got the information about each of them to activate the healing energy. This was the psychic discovery of an ancient method.

The Five Miracles

Following this, he is said to have experienced what is traditionally known as the five miracles, as told by Hawayo Takata. While the authenticity of these stories is somewhat questionable today but we feel they are still worth being told.

1.   When he stood to throw away the last stone, he realised that he felt sturdy. There was no pain, fatigue or hunger, despite not having eaten for 21 days. He felt refreshed and energised and thought to himself, 'This is a miracle'.

2.   While hurrying down the mountain he stubbed his toe and instinctively put his hands on it. His hands became hot and the toe was healed.

3.   On reaching the plain, he went to a house that served pilgrims and asked for a full meal. Though not wise after twenty- one days fasting on water but he ate it without discomfort.

4.   The woman who served the meal to Usui was suffering from toothache. Placing his hands on the sides of her face, he healed her pain.

5.   On his return to the monastery, he was told that the director was in bed with an arthritis attack and severe backache. He placed his hand on his back and narrated the story of his meditation. When he finished narrating the story, the monk exclaimed with surprise that the pain did not exist any longer.

Usui lived for several years in the slums of Kyoto, healing in the town's beggars' quarter. Each person was asked to start a new life after he got healed.

However, after a while, Usui found the beggars returning. When he asked them why, they told him that begging was an easier life as they could fill their stomachs without struggling.

Discouraged and disappointed, he left the slums. On meditating for an answer, he realised that he had assumed that they wanted to be healed - they hadn't asked him for healing, and he had healed them for free, due to which they didn't appreciate its value. This incident would change his attitude toward healing in the future.

During his lifetime, Mikao Usui taught Reiki to more than 2000 people, and initiated seventeen Masters. He died on March 9, 1926 at the age of 62, in Fukuyama.

Chujiro Hayashi

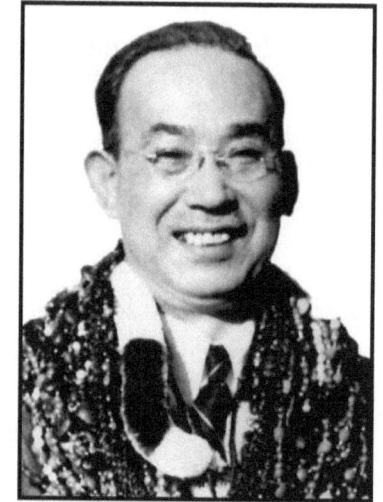

Mikao Usui became a pilgrim traversing Japan on foot. He would walk through the streets of Kyoto with a torch in his hands. When asked why he was carrying a lit torch in broad daylight, he would ask the people if they wanted to know how to bring light, health and happiness in their lives.

Chujiro Hayashi met Mikao Usui when he was holding a lamp at a street corner, announcing his lecture in a nearby temple that evening, to those who asked. A naval commander with the naval reserve, Chujiro Hayashi came from a well-educated and a well to do family. He was impressed with Dr. Usui's sincerity and wisdom, and agreed to accompany him on his travels. He received Reiki Master's training from Mikao Usui in 1925.

Hayashi used the knowledge to open a healing clinic in Tokyo and developed a complex set of hand positions suitable for clinical use of the system. His clinic employed a method of healing that required several practitioners' work on one patient at the same time to maximize the flow of energy. Apart from changing the focus of the system to fit a 'medical' model, Hayashi also introduced a system of 'degrees' in his classes.

Chujiro Hayashi trained teams of Reiki practitioners, both men and women, including sixteen Masters in his lifetime.

Hawayo Takata

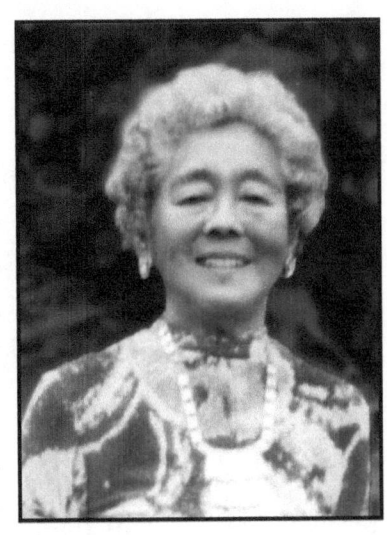

Hawayo Takata was born on December 24, 1900 to a pineapple cutter's family in the island of Kauai, Hawaii. She was too small and frail for plantation work. After her schooling, she lived at the plantation as a housekeeper and bookkeeper. She married the plantation's accountant Saichi Takata, in 1917. They had a happy marriage and two daughters together.

After Saichi Takata died of a heart attack in 1930, Hawayo Takata developed nervous breakdown and severe physical problems. She had a gall bladder disease that required surgery, but had a respiratory condition with breathing difficulties that made the use of anaesthetic dangerous for her.

As her health deteriorated, she was told that she would not live without surgery, but surgery could kill her. She visited her parents in Tokyo and entered the Maeda Medical hospital in Akaska.

In addition to gallstones, she was diagnosed with appendicitis and a tumour. The night before the surgery and on the operating table while being prepared for the anaesthetic, she heard a voice saying, 'The operation is not necessary.'

A Way Out

Hawayo Takata asked the surgeon if there was another way for her to heal. He replied, 'Yes, if you can stay in Japan long enough for it,' and told her about Chujiro Hayashi's clinic. The surgeon's sister, who had been healed by Hayashi's healers and had taken Reiki training, took her to Hayashi's clinic.

Takata was completely healed in body, mind and spirit after spending four months at the clinic. She wished to be trained in Reiki, but was refused as she was a foreigner and Hayashi didn't want the practice of Reiki healing to leave Japan. Eventually, due to the intervention of the Maeda hospital surgeon, Hayashi relented. In 1936 Hawayo Takata received her Reiki I training and she joined the team of healers that worked at Hayashi's clinic. In 1937, she returned to Hawaii after receiving Reiki II training.

The Call

Chujiro Hayashi visited Takata in Hawaii in 1938 and she received her Reiki III training. Hayashi announced Hawayo Takata as a Master/ Teacher. He insisted that she should not give away training without charge.

During the war in 1941, Chujiro Hayashi was asked to join army but as a healer he could not bear the thought of killing others. He could foresee that the clinic would be closed and all involved with Reiki would perish. He did not want Reiki to be totally lost. So he summoned Hawayo Takata psychically and made her his successor. On May 10, 1941, in the presence of his students including Takata, Chujiro Hayashi stopped his own heart by psychic means and died.

Hawayo Takata brought Reiki first to Hawaii, then to mainland United States, and finally to Canada and Europe. She died on December 12, 1980. She always charged her students. Takata came to feel that it was indeed necessary and that people who didn't pay for learning didn't value or use it.

Since Takata's death, Reiki has gone through many changes in the West. Phyllis Furumoto, Takata's successor and granddaughter has been named the Grand Master of Usui Traditional Reiki. Usui Traditional Reiki is also called Usui Reiki Ryoho.

After Takata's death in 1980, a split occurred between Reiki methods, with one group following "Reiki Alliance" lead by Phyllis Furumoto, and another group lead by Ms. Barbara Ray, the American International Reiki Association Inc. (AIRA). Both are based in the USA.

The Emerging Roots of Reiki

At the Saihoji Temple in the Suginami district of Tokyo, a memorial dedicated to Usui Sensei ('Sensei' means teacher or master) was created by the Usui Shiki Reiki Ryoho shortly after Usui Sensei's transition. This is the organization, which Usui Sensei started to promote the practice and teaching of Reiki.

According to the traditional story, all members of this group died in the war or had stopped using Reiki and Hawayo Takata was the only remaining teacher of the Usui system in the world. But as verified by the officials of the Saihoji temple, Usui Shiki Reiki Ryoho has always existed and still exists today. They have been teaching and practicing Reiki in Japan all this time.

According to Arjava Petter, there is no title of "Grand Master" or "Lineage Bearer" in the organization started by Usui Sensei. The person in charge of the organization is the President. Usui Sensei was the first president of the Usui Shiki Reiki Ryoho. Since then there have been five successive presidents. Mr. Kondo, the current president, took over as president when the previous president Ms. Kimiko Koyama passed away at the age of 91.

The inscription on the Usui memorial states it is Usui Sensei's wish that Reiki be spread throughout the world. Reiki was not an oral tradition and both Usui Sensei and Chujiro Hayashi had written material they gave to their students.

Attunements and the practice of Reiki are based more on intuitive guidance and intention than on rigid rules, with Reiki energy being the defining element. The flexibility of the Usui system makes it broad enough to include a wide range of methods and techniques, thus validating the many different styles being practiced today.

Hayashi's gave level I attunements in return for 3 months commitment as unpaid help. They had to work an 8-hour shift once a week for the duration of the commitment. After this time he would offer the better students the second level in return for a further 9-month commitment. Those who completed this had the chance of attaining level 3. After a two-year's further commitment, which involved assisting Hayashi in the classroom, they were taught attunements and were allowed to teach.

A certificate notarised in Honolulu on February 21, 1938 states that Hawayo Takata was made a teacher/master (one of thirteen) of the system; this did not confer the title of Grand Master but simply gave Takata the right to practice and teach the system in the USA.

The entire Usui system is built around the traditional healing system that has been in use for thousands of years in China and surrounding countries. Intent is what guides the system once it is connected to the source. The attunements are just one means of connecting. Reiki can be learned in a single weekend; it is something the body can already do!

The original system before Hayashi had seven hand positions. The patient remained on their back for the whole treatment, which followed the 'top-down' rule of traditional medicine. Hayashi developed this system by experiment and observation. He published a number of papers. It is this document that is the basis of the hand positions that are taught in the West. In the more comprehensive notes in the hands of Tatsumi (he was one of Hayashi's students, and died on October 3, 1996 at an age of 90 years), there is a rigorous 24 position sequence performed by several practitioners at once.

What We Can Learn From History

The two lessons that Dr. Usui learned in the initial days of his Reiki experience hold true even today. These lessons are

1) Heal only those who ask

Taking permission or consent is a very essential lesson we need to learn when healing with Reiki. It is alright to explain to others what Reiki is, and to offer them healing, but they still need to ask first. The exceptions to this rule are inanimate objects, plants, animals, babies and people who are unconscious.

2) Always give Reiki in exchange for something

Reiki should not be given free, for it not only undermines its value, but also discourages people from learning Reiki and healing themselves, thereby creating a dependency. The fee should always be something of value, which could be money, services, or an object.

ABOUT REIKI

Reiki (pronounced ray-kee) written with lower case 'r' is a Japanese compound word meaning Universal Life Force Energy. It is the power that acts and lives in all created matter. 'rei' denotes the universal boundless aspect of this energy while 'ki' is the vital life force energy which flows through all living beings. Many races, cultures and religions have been aware of the existence of an energy that corresponds to the meaning of 'ki'. It is the same as

'*Chi*' in Chinese
'*Prana*' in Sanskrit
'*Mana*' in Hawaiian and
'*Bioplasmic Energy*' by Russian researchers.

Reiki with a capital 'R' is a specific healing support system, which has been passed along from teacher to student for the past hundred years since its rediscovery by Mikao Usui. Usui system of Reiki is a very simple and natural healing method, that works by effectively transferring this Universal Life Force Energy.

In Reiki, we connect with the Universal Life Force Energy which then works automatically to heal a person on all levels. Once a person has been opened up to become a "channel" for Reiki, concentrated Life Energy will flow through his hands of its own accord.

Love, balance, order and harmony are the four master keys of Reiki. Very receptive people often experience Reiki as love. Love is a uniting power that leads us forward to the state of oneness with the whole of creation. The real goal of mankind is to translate this state into reality and to live it out. Love is the original home of the soul, where it returns to be united as a drop with the boundless ocean of being.

To practice Reiki, no special faith or belief is required. Neither do you need education nor experience. It is holistic in its effect. You do not need any tools or equipment.

While practicing Reiki, you can sit, talk, walk, laugh, or read. You can practice Reiki in the morning, noon, evening, night, while travelling, working or watching television.

The Effect of Reiki

Initiation to Reiki does not necessarily turn you into a great healer, wealthy businessman or celebrity. It simply brings out the best in you, intensifies all your capabilities and helps you cope and learn from every situation in life. The overall effect of Reiki is to help bring the body into a perfect balance so that it can heal itself.

Each person responds differently to Reiki. Since it works where the recipient needs it most, no general rule exists. The most common experience is a sense of peace and relaxation, often combined with a pleasant feeling of security and of being enclosed in a fine sheath of energy. Many Reiki recipients begin to relax during treatment and may even fall asleep.

Reiki brings us a decisive step closer to a state of order. One is brought back into a state of unity with the harmony of the Universe. This harmony that is able to reach him in his smallest of cells, makes him whole and healthy again, thus encouraging the natural ability of the patient to heal himself.

With Reiki, a person is healed at all levels- physical, mental, emotional, and spiritual. Reiki is everlasting, instantly available, reliable, soothing and devoid of complications. Reiki helps to raise the level of your vitality for physical and mental health, as well as to enhance spiritual awareness.

Reiki impacts every sphere of your life. It reaches all levels of existence and strives to bring these levels into a state of 'balance'.

Reiki synchronizes and energizes vital body meridians and acupressure points while gently aligning and balancing the major energy centres or 'chakras'. This natural healing system is in perfect harmony with all other healing practices and medical procedures. It is an energy support system that acts in conjunction with all healing practices.

Reiki is greatly beneficial to all life forms- humans, plants, animals and other living forces. It is a consistent and vital means of relieving and releasing stress, tension and hypertension. It is an effective way of creating high level of well- being and reducing cost of health care.

Reiki heals the anxiety associated with diseases and crises, by gently calming the mind and emotions and provides a positive environment for healing. The connection between you and an infinite supply of intelligent, vital life energy releases you from feelings of helplessness and provides a constant and living contact with the Universal Presence.

Reiki energy reduces the side effects of chemotherapy and radiation treatment. It will not prevent the passing over of a person or animal at the designated time, but it eases the process of death. Reiki is a help and comfort for persons grieving over the passing over of their loved ones.

In most congenital birth defects, Reiki is a great blessing and can bring about improvement in even seemingly hopeless conditions.

Similarly, though Reiki may not correct a permanent disability, it helps to make living with the condition as comfortable as possible. Reiki eases the pain, brings relaxation in tense muscles and calms the emotions. Reiki cannot replace an organ removed surgically or an amputated limb, but it will help a person adjust himself to the loss and to new ways of functioning.

Reiki is a very balancing energy and it cannot create an imbalance. It can never cause any harm.

Benefits of Reiki

We can summarize the effects of Reiki as:

1. It brings about deep relaxation.
2. It dissolves energy blockages.
3. It cleanses the body of poisons.
4. It supplies healing Universal Life Force Energy.
5. It increases the frequency of vibration of the body.

Additional effects:

1. It enhances the body's natural ability to heal itself and strengthens the immune system.
2. It vitalizes both body and soul.
3. It re-establishes spiritual equilibrium and mental well-being.
4. It functions on all levels- physical, mental, emotional, spiritual and social.
5. It balances the body's energies.
6. It adjusts itself according to the needs of the recipient.
7. It works with animals and plants.
8. It gives clarity to solve problems.
9. It reduces pain, reduces the side effects of drugs and provides relief in both acute and chronic health problems.

The Five Reiki Principles

Mikao Usui provided five simple Reiki principles for spiritual growth. They should be spoken daily, once in the morning and once in the evening, with intent to incorporate them in day-to-day actions. These principles are:

1. Just for today, I will not anger (stay calm)
2. Just for today, I will not worry (have faith)
3. Just for today, I will be grateful
4. Just for today, I will do my work honestly
5. Just for today, I will be kind to every living thing

Just for today, I will not anger

Remaining calm can have tremendous positive effects on your body. Anger, whether with oneself, others or the world at large creates serious energetic blockages. It is the worst punishment we can give ourselves.

Reiki helps you dissolve blockages caused by anger and accumulated in your body over the years, apart from helping you remain calmer. However, the effort has to be continuous.

Anger is caused when we feel that we have been wronged or when someone does something that we would not have done, had we been in his/ her place. We can eliminate these feelings by reminding ourselves that we never really see the true picture and everyone has a reason behind their deeds.

Replace anger with love, and you will experience peace.

Just for today, stay calm.

Just for today, I will not worry

Concern is very different from worry. While concern for people, events or objects leads us to be proactive and deal with the situation, worry makes us feel helpless, apart from deteriorating our health.

Faith is a very effective antidote for worry. A limitless faith in Reiki or the universe, that whatever happens is for our good alone, and any obstacles in our path are placed there to strengthen us, will help dispel all our worries.

Worry exhausts the mind of a large amount of energy, and a mind free of worry is capable of performing far better and coming up with far more creative ideas and practical solutions.

Letting go of worry, helps the body heal faster.

Just for today, have faith.

Just for today, I will be grateful

We often look at those who have more than we do, and feel unhappy. A simple reversal in this thought process will render our life much happier and content.

A brilliant but blind singer once told me, that sight is the most precious gift man ever got. Those words struck me very deeply. There are millions of disabled people in the world; those who cannot see, hear, talk or have lost a limb. There are so many more who go to bed hungry, on a cold stone floor, with nothing to keep them warm.

When you tend to waste food, think of the malnourished children who are dying of hunger. When you can't buy that costly shirt or dress, remember the cold and unclothed poor. When you crib about your family members, think of those who have no family.

Gratitude is a very powerful emotion and causes changes in both body and mind, helping you become healthier and happier. It is also responsible for bringing greater prosperity in your life.

Be grateful to God for all the miracles in your life. Be grateful for all your problems; let them remind you that if you didn't have the facility, you wouldn't have had the problem at all. An attitude of gratitude lightens your heart and fills your life with joy.

Just for today, I will do my work honestly

Be true and honest to your own conscience and to others. Dishonesty and deceit cause blocks in your progress, and you will receive far lesser than you were destined to. Every temptation is a test, and passing it will take you to the next level of wisdom and energy.

By earning an honest and respectable living, you will open up your life to peace and joy. Working honestly and with all effort is a great opportunity to show gratefulness to the universe for all our gifts. Hard work brings rewards, which enrich your soul.

Just for today, I will be kind to every living thing

Be kind not just to humans, but to animals, plants and non-living objects. A loving outlook in life fills your world with positive energy.

The first step in love is respect. Respect everyone; whether big or small, old or young, and you shall receive respect in return. Allow people their mistakes.

Respect and honour your parents, teachers and elders. If you are open to the lessons you can learn from them, you will gain from their experience and grow wise. Respect children, not just because they are the youth of tomorrow, but also because they are a generation ahead and hence more creative and evolved than you; learning from children keeps us forever youthful and alert. Shower love on everyone and be helpful to all.

LEARNING REIKI

The ability to use Reiki is transferred to the student by the Reiki Master/Teacher through an empowerment within an attunement process or ceremony. It is like a re-awakening of a talent that is lying dormant within you. For some, it may be possible to re-activate this ability on their own but for most, it is much simpler to receive a Reiki attunement.

Because of this, virtually anyone can learn Reiki with no prior experience or ability. The attunement process opens the crown, brow, throat, heart and palm chakras and creates a special link between the student and the Reiki source. The Reiki Master/Teacher then explains and demonstrates its use.

After that, the student simply places her or his hands on someone with the intention of healing and the Reiki energies will automatically flow through the student into the recipient. Because of this unique attunement process, Reiki can be easily taught during one-day class, or less. The Reiki Empowerment is actually a powerful healing experience in itself.

More about Attunement

The attunement/ initiation doesn't give you anything you don't already have. Reiki is cosmic energy, it is what animates us, running through our energy meridians and flowing around us in our electromagnetic field. Each one of us is connected to it from birth. This life force is comparatively very strong in children. With the passage of time, emotional blocks develop in our systems and the flow of Reiki reduces.

The reduction in this rejuvenating energy flow creates a state of uneasiness, a dis-ease. Gradually, due to lack of healing, though mechanical treatment may be there in plenty, this dis-ease becomes a 'disease'.

What happens during an attunement?

During the Reiki attunement, a Reiki Teacher establishes a major re-connection with the source of your spiritual and inner strength. This revitalization overcomes emotional pain and hurt and replaces it with positive happiness. This well-being is reflected on the body as a state of good health. The Reiki attunement uncaps any lid we might have on our natural healing abilities, it dissolves obstructions or interference, and opens the healing channel.

The main difference between having and not having the Reiki attunement is in the quantity and quality in regard to the flow of this vital life force energy. The larger the pipeline, the greater the flow of Reiki energy. After the attunement, the individual is able to receive, utilize and appreciate more the ceaseless flow of this energy.

The attunement is not a healing; it creates a healer. The attunement is what separates other touch healing systems and Reiki. Other systems may use hand positions over the chakras and work with Ki energy but only Reiki has the extraordinary benefit of the attunement process.

Upon receiving the attunement in Reiki I, the receiver becomes a channel for this Universal Healing Energy. Once attuned, all one needs to do to connect with the healing energy is to place his hands upon himself or someone else and it will flow through automatically.

The Usui system consists of three levels or degrees of attunement. Each degree is complete in itself.

Reiki I

Reiki I is said to be a proximity modality. In Reiki I, the attunement itself heals physical level diseases in the person who receives it. One's physical health often changes for the better in the months following the initiation. If practiced properly, this level also re-establishes the lost connection we have with our bodies.

Reiki I primarily is for self-healing, but practitioners can also do healing for someone else who is physically present. Such healing is known as direct healing. The practitioner should be within 2" to 3" of the receiver and he must keep the hands close to the other person's body. The attunement to this level awakens the practitioner. This is like plugging in and turning on a lamp in a house already wired for electricity. The light is switched on when you put your hands down to heal.

A person who is attuned is called a 'Reiki channel', which means he is in a position to channelize the Universal Life Energy for healing on the earth plane. It takes three to four weeks to adjust to the Reiki I attunement. The person may feel spacey or tingly, have intense dreams including past life dreams or experience detoxification symptoms. These can include diarrhea, running nose or increased urination. The person will still feel well. The reactions are because the energy is adjusting and increasing the new healer's capacity to channel it.

More energy is entering the aura than before and the aura and chakras are clearing. If the process gets uncomfortable, healing oneself or another balances the energy and decreases the sensations.

So, for twenty-one days, one must do as many healing sessions as possible, including a daily self -healing.

Optimally, one should use First Degree at least three months before proceeding to Second Degree (if not longer) and then wait a minimum of three years before considering Third Degree.

Reiki I is in no way to be considered inferior to Reiki II or the higher degrees. There is only a difference in the quantum and capability of energy available, not the quality.

Can the Reiki channel feel the flow of energy?

We cannot generalize this. Many people experience heat, cold, vibrations, or see colours or symbols while giving or receiving Reiki treatment and while getting attuned. Whether a Reiki channel feels the energy flow or not, once he is attuned by a qualified teacher, energy flows through his hands when he lays his hands on himself or somebody else with an intention to heal.

Why do some people have sensations, while others do not?

One reason is that these are very subtle sensations. Usually a person expects something drastic to happen and in that expectation, these subtle sensations go unnoticed. So even if he felt heat/ cold, he will tend to attribute it to the temperature or breeze in the room.

Another reason is the spiritual level of the person. If one has been in the habit of listening to his inner voice, he can appreciate the changes occurring in the body during Reiki treatment and Reiki attunement.

But this cannot be generalized, it can be the opposite also. Like a person who never had any spiritual exposure, when a sudden rush of energy enters his body, it is a unique experience for him and he feels it with full impact. This can be compared to the opening of a window in a room that has been closed for some time. When the window is opened suddenly, the wind enters the room with force and it is very palpable.

At the same time, a person who leads a very worldly life, never devoting time to spiritual and philosophical aspects, can be compared to one who always eats food that is highly spicy. Such a person may not appreciate the flavour of vegetables if he eats them without spices.

Reiki is not a hurricane that will turn around your life in a jiffy. It is like a mild breeze, which is going to change your life in each and every sphere, silently, slowly, and definitely.

I am not so sensitive, what do I do?

In all scientific experiments, we proceed with a hypothesis. We start with a belief and do the scientific experiments, sometimes for years together, to either prove or disprove the hypothesis. Similarly, you have to start with the hypothesis that Reiki is going to heal you. For three months, note every change that occurs in your life, not only in the physical aspect, but also in all spheres of your life. For example, some problem that has been worrying you for quite some time suddenly gets solved. Or some person, whom you have wanted to contact, appears.

Initially, you will be tempted to believe that they are just coincidences. Soon however, you will realise that the co-incidences are too many to be attributed to chance. At some point, you realize and acknowledge that Reiki has started healing you and improving your life in every way.

In the modern era, we have endless material things to help us improve our lifestyle. Reiki, on the other hand, improves our life. It will take you beyond material pleasures, into dizzy heights of true enjoyment.

Reiki II

During the Second Degree class, you are taught three symbols or keys that help to focus your mind so that it can send Reiki energy beyond time and space. These keys unlock the Reiki power to those who have received the Second Degree initiations.

The Second level initiation provides a quantum leap in vibratory level, about four times greater than the First.

Second Degree attunements work more directly on the etheric body and tend to stimulate development of the intuitive centre. It focuses on emotional, mental and karmic healing in the person who receives the attunement.

After the attunement, old emotions, unhealed former situations, past lives, and negative mental patterns resurface to be fully healed at last. This can take as long as six months to complete and though not always comfortable, the process is positive and necessary.

Reiki II attunement adds considerable power to direct healing sessions. Now the practitioner can heal those who are not physically near him and also send energy to incidents and occasions in the past, present or future.

Reiki III

Traditionally Reiki III was meant for Masters only. Today, the energy of Reiki III is also available as Reiki III A degree, without the Master's knowledge of attunement so that one may progress further spiritually without taking on the commitment of the Master.

It is not necessary for most Reiki channels. One may consider this step on reaching maturity in Reiki and in life.

Reiki I and II Degrees empower you to create abundance in your life in all areas. Reiki III is meant for furthering the inner detachment from all material issues, which start manifesting with advancement in Reiki training.

This attunement again amplifies the vibratory level. The attunement involves spiritual level energy and achieves spiritual healing in the person receiving it.

Detoxification

A 21-day cleansing process follows Reiki attunement in each of the three degrees. You have read that everything is composed of energy i.e., everything has a vibration. The emotions and negative blocks that are stored in our physical and etheric bodies have a lower vibratory rate than loving and positive thoughts.

During Reiki attunement, there is a sudden increase in the rate of vibrations in our body. This loosens the dense negative energy within our body, which is out of tune with the positive vibrations created by the attunement.

The adjusted vibration releases old stored up emotions and memories. It takes time for the adjustments to be effective. Approximately three days are taken for the energy to move through each of the seven main chakras.

Although the opening of the Reiki channel occurs between the heart chakra and the crown chakra, other three major chakras are equally important and go through a corresponding adjustment in the vibratory rate.

During the cleansing period, you may experience strange feelings, emotional changes, various dreams, physical changes such as detoxification, and an old habit or favourite food losing its importance in your life. Some reactions may be unpleasant at first. But by accepting them instead of resisting, and without attaching undue concern, each one will simply pass away.

For the stored toxins in the body to be released easily during this period, it is important to drink a lot of water.

It is highly recommended that you keep a diary during this process to record the changes that occur. Develop a habit of giving yourself Reiki treatments before you fall asleep at night and first thing after you wake up in the morning.

Continuous self-healing practice after the initial cleansing process, further refines your energy and helps your spiritual growth. As old undesirable feelings and concepts get released, you will begin to feel the attitude of gratitude flow naturally in your life, creating a greater level of abundance in all areas in your life..

The Power-Centres of Our Body:
CHAKRAS

'Chakra' is a Sanskrit word meaning wheel, and chakras in our body are in fact a whirl of energy. It is through the chakras that the energy field of our body breathes. They are like tornadoes or small vortexes.

Chakras determine a person's physical, psychological, emotional, as well as spiritual well-being. The chakras correspond exactly, in number and position to the endocrine glands in our body. Each chakra has a related colour, crystal, oil, sound, exercise and food.

The etheric and physical bodies are connected, as are the chakras and endocrine glands. The etheric body is an energy body of very fine vibrations, totally enveloping the physical body. It absorbs the finer energies from the environment and transduces this energy through the chakras into the physical body via the endocrine glands.

If there is an imbalance in the chakras, the endocrine system can go out of balance, which in turn affects the hormonal balance.

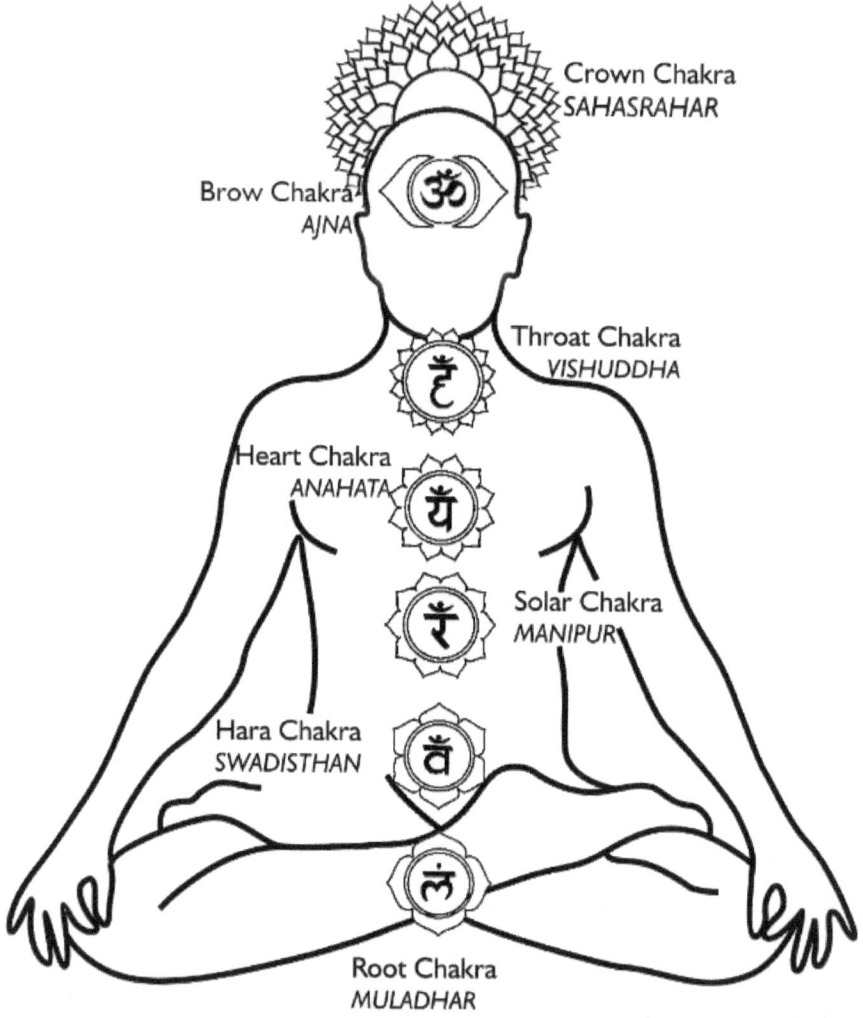

Crown Chakra
SAHASRAHAR

Brow Chakra
AJNA

Throat Chakra
VISHUDDHA

Heart Chakra
ANAHATA

Solar Chakra
MANIPUR

Hara Chakra
SWADISTHAN

Root Chakra
MULADHAR

This can have a powerful effect on the person's moods and emotions. Conversely, if an imbalance occurs in the endocrine system, it will put the chakra system out of balance.

Reiki energy is absorbed by both systems simultaneously, making it an excellent modality for creating balance in the chakras and the endocrine glands. The body has seven major chakras. All the chakras are of equal importance.

The information listed below is not intended for the use of beginners of Reiki, but only after a little practice. This information can be used to supplement your healing when you feel that a chakra is particularly deficient in energy and needs more healing than usual.

The energy needs of chakras vary day to day, and there is no need to refer to this information for small differences in energy needs. However, if and when you encounter a severe lack or a block in energies, you may resort to this information to help you with further healing.

First chakra

Base or **Root chakra** is located at the base of the spine (coccyx). This chakra is the grounding point through which the Divine Essence takes up its permanent residence in the body, superimposing the consciousness of the crown chakra and the unconditional love of the heart. It assists in letting go of all unwanted concepts.

Root chakra is the source of self-preservation and survival. It represents the evolutionary life force and is associated with our sense of belonging in the world and our surroundings. It symbolizes the physical plane of existence both the earth and your physical body.

When this chakra is clear and unblocked, positive energy can flow from it freely. Such a person is likely to experience a solid feeling of safety and security in day-to-day life. One knows at a deeper level that loved ones are truly there for you. A person with a strong root chakra generally feels grounded and understands that his life's foundation is solid. He isn't apt to be as swayed by life's small ups and downs as many people are.

Disturbance in the root chakra effectively leaves one without 'roots'. This may result in feelings of loneliness, fear for safety and a disconnection from other people. One is also likely to feel ungrounded, lacking a strong connection to the earth or the body.

Sanskrit Name : Muladhara
Meaning   : Root
Location   : Pelvis, perineum
Element   : Earth
Sense   : Smell
Glands   : Sexual and Adrenal
Areas   : Legs, hips, spinal bones, male sexual organs, large
                intestine.
Function   : Grounding
Malfunction   : Obesity, haemorrhoids, constipation, sciatica,
                degenerative arthritis
Enemy   : Fear
Food   : Proteins, meat
Colour   : Red
Stones   : Agate, Ruby
Sound   : Lam

More about the Root Chakra

Central issues: Survival, stability, acceptance, self-preservation, deep-rootedness, perception, grounding, fear and safety

Excessive: Sluggish, lazy, tired, monotony, obesity, overeating, hoarding, materialism, greed, Fear of change, addiction to security

Deficient: Fearful, anxious, restless, lack of discipline, underweight, financial difficulty, chronic disorganization

Balanced: Good health, vitality, well grounded, sense of trust in the world, feeling safe and secure, stability, prosperity, ability to relax

Physical Dysfunctions: Frequent illness, disorders of the bowel, large intestine, bones, teeth, problems with legs, feet, base of spine (chronic lower back pain, sciatica), eating disorders, depression, immune-related disorders, skin problems; lack of energy

Addictions: Food, gambling, shopping, work

Traumas and abuses: Birth trauma, abandonment, physical neglect, poor physical bonding with the mother, malnourishment, feeding difficulty, major illness or surgery, physical abuse, inherited traumas (eg. war, poverty, etc.)

Spiritual challenge: How well we manage our physical world

Healing Strategy: Physical activity, lots of touch, massage, reconnect with the body, grounding, Hatha yoga, look at earliest childhood relationship to mother, reclaim your right to be here

Feeding Your Root Chakra

Root vegetables: carrots, potatoes, parsnips, radishes, beets, onions, garlic, etc.

Protein-rich foods: eggs, meats, beans, tofu, peanuts

Spices: horseradish, hot paprika, chives, cayenne, pepper

Exercise: stomping your feet, marching, squats

Second chakra

Hara or Sacral chakra is located at the base of the spine at the level of the coccyx, and pubic bone. When healing this chakra with Reiki, we heal between the pubic bone and the naval point (3 finger-widths below the navel). This chakra represents honour and is the seat of creativity. It is also the place of false ego (*ahankara*). This chakra is located at the sacrum, which is the densest bone in the spinal column.

A person with a strong hara values others and is secure in relationships. This chakra often offers us the opportunity to let go of our "control issues" and find balance in our lives. It helps us recognize that acceptance and rejection are not the only options in relationships. Bringing about life changes through personal choices is a theme of second chakra energy.

A person with a closed second chakra can appear lifeless. This is because it can cut one off from emotions, and one may feel removed from an interest in sexuality. On the other hand, if the second chakra is excessively open, emotions can sometimes rule one's being, creating an unbalanced system overall. Rejuvenation, regeneration and revitalization of the physical body can be stimulated from here.

When the hara region is healthy, we can live with ourselves in harmony and peace - with the parts of ourselves that we do not like, such as failures, alcoholic tendencies, flirtatious nature, submissive nature etc.,

All these fragments of us reside at the hara, weakening our abilities to achieve and create. Past emotional hurts thought over, meditated upon and consequent pain — all accumulate here, damaging our purpose of life.

Sanskrit Name : Svadisthana
Meaning   : Sweetness
Location   : Lower part of abdomen
Element   : Water
Sense   : Taste
Glands   : Ovaries and testicles
Areas   : Womb, genitals, bladder, circulatory system, intestines, colon, skin, female sexual organs
Function   : Desire, pleasure, sexuality.
Malfunction : Impotence, frigidity, uterine, bladder and kidney trouble, stiff lower back, blocked creativity, allergies
Enemy   : Guilt
Food   : Liquid
Colour   : Orange
Stones   : Coral, topaz, opal
Sound   : Vam

More about the Hara Chakra

Central issues: Sexuality, emotions, financial, creativity, codes of honour and ethics

Excessive: Addiction to substance/ sex, emotional dependency, excessively sensitive, strong emotions, invasion of others, seductive manipulation, obsessive attachment

Deficient: Poor social skills, lack of desire/ passion/ excitement, frigidity, fear of sex, denial of pleasure, fear of change, rigidity

Balanced: Graceful movements; emotional intelligence; ability to experience pleasure; nurture of self and others; ability to change; healthy boundaries

Physical Dysfunctions: Sexual dysfunctions, Ob/Gyn. problems, dysfunctions of reproductive organs, spleen, urinary system; loss of appetite for food, sex, life; chronic lower back pain, sciatica;

Addictions: Alcohol, sex, heroin

Traumas and abuses: Sexual, emotional abuse, neglect, rejection, emotional manipulation, physical abuse, alcoholic families, denial of child's feelings

Spiritual challenges: Negative one-to-one control patterns need to be confronted

Healing Strategy: Movement therapies; emotional release; assign healthy pleasures; develop sensate intelligence

Feeding Your Sacral Centre

Sweet fruits: melons, mangos, strawberries, passion fruit, oranges, coconut, etc.

Honey & Nuts: almonds, walnuts, etc.

Spices: cinnamon, vanilla, carob, sweet paprika, sesame seeds, caraway seeds

Exercise: circular pelvis movements, pelvic thrusts

Third chakra

Solar plexus chakra is associated with personal power and is located where the sternum ends, the ribs separate and the abdominal cavity (3 finger-widths above the navel). Some Sanskrit texts mention the Manipura chakra as being located at the navel, on the spine. In this case, a secondary chakra called Surya is shown in the solar plexus.

This chakra functions in harmony with the heart and represents one's ability to honour and accept the self. Rich in ganglia and interconnected neurons, the solar plexus is the largest autonomic nerve centre in the abdominal cavity and hence is also known as the second brain.

People who are empowered have high positive energy emanating from their third chakras. Knowing that you can move things forward in your life in order to learn, grow, and live well is closely related to having a clear third chakra. Individual charisma is also generated in this energetic region. A person with a strong solar chakra is apt to treat oneself with kindness, to forgive personal mistakes rather than dwell on them unnecessarily.

A blocked solar chakra leads to a lack of trust in personal perceptions and decisions, along with lack of energy, fatigue, and a yearning to be quiet and shut down. Confrontations with others can be very hard to initiate and tolerate. It can also lead to problems in building and sustaining interpersonal relationships based on equality.

Sanskrit Name : Manipura
Meaning   : Jewel
Location   : Solar Plexus
Element   : Fire
Sense   : Sight
Glands   : Pancreas, adrenals

Areas	: Digestive system, muscles, liver, gall bladder, stomach, pancreas.
Function	: Will power, confidence, seat of emotions, spiritual/ psychic site
Malfunction	: Ulcer, diabetes, hypoglycaemia.
Enemy	: Shame
Food	: Carbohydrates
Colour	: Yellow or yellow gold
Stones	: Topaz
Sound	: Ram

More about the Solar Plexus Chakra

Central issues: Power, self-esteem, self-image, energy, will, responsibility

Excessive: Overly aggressive, dominating, controlling, blaming, arrogance, manipulative, power hungry, stubbornness, hyperactivity, excessively ambitious and competitive

Deficient: Low energy, weak will, poor self-esteem, passive, sluggish, fearful, poor self-discipline, emotionally and physically cold, victim mentality, blaming of others, unreliable, poor digestion

Balanced: Feeling of tranquillity and inner harmony, self-acceptance, respect for the nature and emotions of others, feeling of unity with the rest of humanity, responsible, reliable, confidence, spontaneity, sense of humour, able to meet challenges

Physical Dysfunctions: Arthritis, digestive disorders, ulcers, colon and intestinal problems, anorexia or bulimia, pancreatitis, diabetes, gallstone, allergies, problems with the stomach and liver

Addictions: Amphetamines, cocaine, caffeine, work, anger

Traumas and abuses: Shaming, authoritarianism, physical abuse, fear of punishment, dangerous environment, age inappropriate responsibilities, inherited shame from parents

Spiritual challenges: Maturation of the ego

Healing Strategy: Risk taking, grounding, emotional contact, deep relaxation, stress control, vigorous exercise, sit-ups, psychotherapy (release or contain anger, build ego strength, work on shame issues, strengthen will)

Feeding Your Solar Plexus Chakra

Granola and Grains: pastas, breads, cereal, rice, flax seed, sunflower seeds, etc.

Dairy: milk, cheeses, yogurt

Spices: ginger, mints (peppermint, spearmint, etc.), chamomile, turmeric, cumin, fennel

Exercise: belly dancing, doing the twist, hoola hooping

Fourth chakra

Heart chakra is located near the heart and is associated with a gradual increasing of consciousness, as it sits between the lower three and upper three chakras. It represents higher emotions, such as love, tenderness, and compassion. It is the seat of unconditional love, and is adversely affected by stress.

People with a strong heart chakra are open, loving, and compassionate to those around them and are very accepting of people for who they are. They possess an emotional maturity and depth that allows them to empathize with others. Whether interacting with strangers or loved ones, the heart chakra conveys the kind of true compassion that can set others at ease.

A disconnection from the heart and emotions leads to a closing of the heart chakra, often resulting in low energy and shallow breathing.. Emotionally, it is associated with feeling wounded or victimized. Often this will be due to trying to work out past problems. It may also be difficult to protect oneself from emotional harm because one tends to feel raw and vulnerable.

Sanskrit Name : Anahata
Meaning : Unstruck (Sound that is made without 2 objects colliding)
Location : Heart
Element : Air
Sense : Touch
Glands : Thymus
Areas : Lungs, heart, arm, hands, shoulders, blood, thymus, knees.
Function : Love, compassion, peace, harmony, contentment, balance, forgiveness
Malfunction : Asthma, high blood pressure, heart disease, breast cancer, arthritis

Enemy   : Grief
Food   : Fruits and Vegetables
Colour   : Green or pink
Stones   : Emerald
Sound   : Yam

More about the Heart Chakra

Central issues: Love, unconditional love, self-love, forgiveness, relationships, intimacy, devotion, depression and loneliness

Excessive: Demanding, jealousy, co-dependency, poor boundaries, overly sacrificing, possessive

Deficient: Antisocial, withdrawn, cold, shy, critical, judgmental, intolerant, loneliness, depression, fear of intimacy/ relationships, lack of empathy, narcissism, bitter

Balanced: Compassionate, loving, self-loving, empathetic, peaceful, balanced, good immune system

Physical Dysfunctions: Disorders of the heart, lungs, thymus, breast, arms, asthma, allergy, circulation problems, immune system deficiency, tension between shoulder blades

Addictions: Tobacco (smoking), sugar, love, marijuana

Traumas and Addictions: rejection, abandonment, loss, shaming, constant criticism, abuses to lower chakras, unacknowledged grief, divorce, death, conditional love, loveless environment, sexual and physical abuse, betrayal

Spiritual challenges: To learn compassion, the value of forgiveness, unconditional love

Healing Strategy: Self-discovery, co-dependency, work, forgiveness, inner child work, work with arms, reaching out, taking in, breathing exercise

Feeding Your Heart Chakra

Leafy vegetables: spinach, kale, dandelion greens, etc.

Air vegetables: broccoli, cauliflower, cabbage, celery, squash, etc

Liquids: green teas

Spices: basil, sage, thyme, cilantro, parsley

Exercise: push ups, swimming (breast stroke), hugging yourself

Fifth chakra

Throat chakra is located at the throat and is associated with sound in general, and in specific with acts of communication, including speaking the truth or finding creative ways for self-expression. It represents honesty and truth.

It is the centre for purification, creativity and all forms of expression. A person with a strong throat chakra communicates effectively at all levels, is a good listener and has good connection between the internal and external self and between body and mind.

A strong throat chakra brings a burning need to speak the truth without fearing the consequences. It makes one treat people with respect, and act with integrity. This chakra is also associated with personal will.

When it is in a state of balance, one does not tend to fight life's natural path, but align more easily with divine will. During such periods, one is likely to feel that things are going one's way, rather than having to fight the current in order to reach one's goals.

When the throat chakra is too open, one may talk too much and be a poor listener.

When the throat chakra is too weak, one may be afraid to express opinions and personal truths. One will often feel unsure about what to say. Personal will can seem non-existent. Disruptions in the throat chakra cause people to blame everyone else when things go wrong, and take all credit when things go right.

Sanskrit Name : Vishuddhi
Meaning : Purified
Location : Throat
Element : Ether
Sense : Hearing
Glands : Thyroid
Areas : Neck, shoulders, arms and hands, thyroid, throat and mouth, parathyroid
Function : Creativity, communication, power of speech, harmony, expression
Malfunction : Sore throat, lack of communication, thyroid problems.
Enemy : Lies
Food : Fruit
Colour : Blue
Stones : Turquoise, aquamarine
Sound : Ham

More about the Throat Chakra

Central issues: Communication, self-expression, self-discipline, speaking one's truth

Excessive: Too much talking, talking as a defence, inability to listen, gossiping, interruptions, over-extended, stuttering

Deficient: Fear of speaking, small, weak voice, difficulty in putting feelings into words, shyness, tone deaf, poor rhythm

Balanced: Good listener, resonant voice, good sense of timing and rhythm, clear communication, lives creatively

Physical Dysfunctions: Raspy throat, chronic sore throat, mouth ulcers, gum difficulties, scoliosis, laryngitis, swollen glands, thyroid problems, headaches, neck or shoulder pain, ear infections / problems

Addictions: Opiates, marijuana

Traumas and abuses: Lies, secrets, verbal abuse, constant yelling, excessive criticism (blocks creativity), authoritarian parents, alcoholic, chemical dependent family

Spiritual challenges: To recognize that your strength of will is measured not by how well you exert your will over others, but how well you control yourself. Conscious self-control and discipline means living according to the truth that every thought you have is either a potential act of grace or a potential weapon. Right thought leads to right speech leads to right acting.

Healing Strategy: Learn communication skills, letter writing, inner child communication, practice silence (excessive), storytelling, singing, chanting, toning, release voice, and loosen neck and shoulders

Feeding Your Throat Chakra

Liquids in general: water, fruit juices, herbal teas

Tart or tangy fruits: lemons, limes, grapefruit, kiwi

Other tree growing fruits: apples, pears, plums, peaches, apricots

Spices: salt, lemon grass

Exercise: gargling with salt water, singing, screaming

Sixth chakra

Brow chakra is located in the lower brain and at the third eye, which is between the eyebrows and is known as the eye of the soul. It is associated both with light and with psychic abilities and represents our ability to see and really know truth, being able look past superficialities to see life's core realities.

This chakra provides a source of inner knowing, as well as an objective reflection of how things are. By being focused on a commitment to truth and flexibility of thought, people with clear sixth chakras usually have a sense of life's realities that surpasses usual conscious barriers. As a result, the sixth chakra is connected with higher levels of wisdom and a level disposition. It also makes people with strong brow chakras more objective than many people. At times, this positive flow of energy from your sixth chakra can even heighten psychic powers, helping one to know the unknowable.

When the brow chakra is balanced and strong, one will usually have a higher level of intuition than most people. One will also be more accepting of the people and events rather being judgmental. One does not feel threatened or personally accused by others' beliefs, thereby escaping the pain that most people inflict upon themselves. This also helps to become very objective about criticism, and helps separate constructive and destructive criticism.

A problem in the brow chakra will create a problem in seeing the big picture of events that are unfolding in life. The truth of matters can be dwarfed in details, and confusion increases. One tends to overlook the subtler forces in any situation because the attention is focused on literal details. One is also likely to be judge people and events quite harshly.

Sanskrit Name : Ajna
Meaning   : The centre of command
Location   : Centre of Forehead – between the eyes
Element   : Light
Sense   : Intuition
Glands   : Pituitary
Areas   : Eyes
Function   : Intuition and wisdom
Malfunction : Blindness, headaches, nightmares, eye strain,
                blurred vision
Enemy   : Illusion
Food   : Fast
Colour   : Indigo
Stones   : Amethyst
Sound   : Aum

More about the Brow Chakra

Central issue: Intuition, imagination, ability to see one's life clearly, use of the mind/intellect

Excessive: Hallucination, nightmares, obsessions, delusions, difficulty concentrating, headaches

Deficient: Poor vision and memory, insensitivity, lack of imagination, difficulty visualizing, difficulty seeing the future, can't remember dreams, denial

Balanced: Intuitive, perceptive, imaginative, good memory, able to visualize, able to think symbolically, able to remember dreams

Physical Dysfunctions: Headaches, eye and ear disease, nose and sinus problems, facial nerve problems, nightmares, brain tumour, stroke, neurological disturbances, seizures, full spinal difficulty, learning disabilities

Addictions: Hallucinogens, marijuana

Traumas and abuses: Frightening environment (war, violence), what you see does not go with what you are told, invalidation of intuition and psychic occurrences

Spiritual challenges: Pride and the ability to make judgments. The spiritual lessons relate to insight and intuition, to seeing beyond the visible.

Healing Strategy: Meditation, visual stimulation, create visual art, colouring and drawing, working with memory, dream work, hypnosis, guided visualization, past life regression therapy

Feeding Your Brow Chakra

Dark blue fruits: blueberries, red grapes, black berries, etc.

Liquids: red wines and grape juice

Spices: lavender, poppy seed

Exercise: visualization, remote viewing, lucid dreaming

Seventh chakra

Crown chakra is located at the crown of the head, but it is connected with the entire muscular system, the skeletal system, the skin, and nervous system. It is the highest seat of consciousness and is associated with thought. It signifies our relationship to all things and the unity of everything. This chakra also symbolizes self-knowledge and spiritual consciousness.

The seventh chakra is associated with a more profound spiritual connectedness than the other six chakras are. This chakra is the seat of higher wisdom and the energy that comes from it. The seventh chakra is thought to give access to the infinite intelligence that exists in the universe and is our key to opening the door to it.

This chakra allows for self-expression on higher spiritual levels and is associated with the pineal gland, the gland that produces visions in dreams. When asking the question, "Who am I, really?" you are tapping into the energy of your seventh chakra.

For people who possess powerful seventh chakra energy, the spiritual world can be as real as the physical environment that exists all around. At times, the connection with a higher power can also help to transcend the common confusion of life's day-to-day happenings to feel truly at peace.

However, on other occasions, being so spiritually inclined may leave one vulnerable to pangs of confusion or doubt; these are times when faith is shaken. Ultimately such difficult periods will usually only serve to make one's spiritual alliance stronger, furthering one along life's path.

A person with a blocked crown chakra can feel cut off from spirituality and fears of the spiritual aspects of life can be magnified. It can also amount to the inability to gain closure on unfinished business. Most of all, lack of flow in the seventh chakra leads to an inability to live in the present. People with blocked seventh chakra energy seem to always be either revisiting their past or looking ahead into the future.

Sanskrit Name : Sahasrahara
Meaning   : Thousand Petals
Location   : Top of the head
Element   : Thought
Sense   : Psychological state is bliss
Glands   : Pineal
Areas   : Cerebral cortex, right eye, upper brain.
Function   : Thought, understanding, spiritual will, divine wisdom.
Malfunction : Depression, apathy, senility, alienation, confusion, migraines, asthma, inability to learn/ comprehend
Enemy   : Attachment
Food   : Fast
Colour   : Violet
Stones   : Diamond, clear quartz
Sound   : Ahhhh

More about the Crown Chakra

Central issue: Awareness, spiritual search for meaning, issues of karma and grace, grace bank account, spiritual awakening, divine discontent

Excessive: Over-intellectualization, spiritual addiction, confusion, dissociation from body

Deficient: Spiritual cynicism, learning difficulties, rigid belief systems, apathy, materialism, greed, domination

Balanced: Sense of spiritual connection, open-minded, wisdom and mastery, broad understanding, intelligent, thoughtful, aware, ability to perceive, analyze and assimilate information

Physical Dysfunctions: Energetic disorders, mystical depression, coma, migraines, brain tumours, amnesia, chronic exhaustion not linked to physical disorder, sensitivity to light, sound and other environmental factors

Addictions: Religion, spiritual practices

Traumas and Addictions: Spiritual abuse, forced religiosity, blind obedience, misinformation, lies, withheld information, invalidation of one's beliefs

Spiritual challenges: Hope and faith, spiritual conscience. Spiritual quests and questions of your life:
For what purpose was I born?
What is truth?
What is the deeper meaning of life? Can I find that?
Failure to hear and respond to these questions can lead to anxiety and depression.

Healing Strategy: Re-establish physical, emotional, spirit connection, spiritual discipline and meditation; examine belief systems and goal setting

Feeding Your Crown Chakra

Air: fasting / detoxing

Incense & Smudging Herbs: sage, copal, myrrh, frankincense, and juniper

Incense and smudging herbs are ritually inhaled through the nostrils or can be smoked through a ceremony pipe for purification purposes.

Exercise: prayer, meditation

HEALING YOURSELF

The only person who can heal someone is himself. Healing can and does happen in your own body. A Reiki channel's role is simple; he merely channels Reiki energy, which the patient uses in any way that is best suited for his needs.

Here, healing is a three-way agreement. The Reiki channel, the patient, and the Universal Energy source are jointly involved in a Reiki healing. Between the source at one end, and the patient at the other, the Reiki channel (healer) volunteers to become a medium, a channel in between them. Therefore, without the patient's consent, as also his participation in the healing process, no healing can take place.

Reiki is never sent; it is drawn through the channel. If I lay hands on you to do a treatment, you will draw appropriate amounts of energy to the low-energy areas of your body. I am never drained in the process. At the same time, you do not take on any of my negative energy or blocks, because the Reiki passes through a purified channel in my body, opened by the attunement.

Researchers at Stanford, using highly sensitive instruments, which measure the flow of energy forces entering the body, determined that Reiki Energy enters the healer through the top of the head (crown chakra) and exits through the hands. Once the Reiki Energy is activated, it seems to flow in a counter clockwise spiral motion, much like the double helix in the DNA.

The Importance

The moment you are attuned by a qualified Reiki Teacher, you become a Reiki channel, i.e., the Universal Life Energy enters your body through the crown chakra and exits through the palm.

Whether you can appreciate the flow of energy or not depends on your sensitivity. Some are able to feel the flow of energy right from the time of attunement as heat, cold or numbness in the palms. Others may not feel the energy flow, even though they see the results of the channelled energy later on.

The amount of energy you can channel initially depends on your spiritual level at the time. Whatever level this may be, it keeps on increasing by constant practice.

For daily self-healing, basic thirteen positions are recommended. You can add more positions as per your intuition. We channel the energy to the seven major chakras. The top most chakra, the crown chakra is given energy once and all other chakras are given energy from the front and back of the body (6+6=12), hence the thirteen basic positions.

The sequence in which you give Reiki to the chakras isn't critical, but it is better to follow an orderly sequence so that no position will be missed out and you don't have to think much to decide the next position. Once you practice the thirteen positions in order, it becomes a habit and the hands automatically move to the next point. Instead of straining to remember the positions to be covered, you can focus on the rise and fall of the energy flow.

Do not cross your arms or legs during Reiki healing as it can interfere with the free flow of energy.

Though Reiki can be done anywhere and at any time, it is good if you can fix a place and time for Reiki sessions. It is like having your lunch at the same time every day. By the time you wash your hands and sit for the meal, your body is ready to accept the food. The mouth starts salivating; the stomach starts secreting acid etc.

The body can receive more powerfully if you adhere to a particular timing. The space where you practice Reiki becomes charged with energy. So practicing at the same time, same place every day improves the efficiency of your practice.

How to hold your hands

The first thing a Reiki channel needs to know is how to hold his hands. Both hands, held palms down, are used in Reiki. Both hands must be on the receiver's body, or held just above it, for the energy to flow through. Fingers and thumbs are extended and held together, and the palms slightly cupped.

The life force energy flows through the chakras in the centres of the palms and the tips of each finger. If for some reason both hands can't be placed on a position, place one hand on the position and the other somewhere else on the receiver's body.

Energy can radiate through hands at other times than during healing sessions. New Reiki channels may report that their hands grow hot at odd times, and this may happen for the first few weeks. When you are sitting close to someone who needs the energy, your hands may heat up. Reiki can also activate when your hands are resting on your own body.

Preparing For Whole Body Reiki

Self-healing sessions can be comfortably done when you are sitting relaxed in a chair. It can also be done in bed the last thing at night or first thing in the morning.

Although Reiki can be done anywhere and at any time, its benefits can be felt the most if certain steps are taken before starting the healing. However, not being able to follow these shouldn't act as a deterrent to a prospective healing session.

Remove Accessories and Shoes

Remove items such as earrings, eyeglasses, watches and belts. The stones (semi-precious or precious), metal rings or chains, etc. attract energies that may interfere with the life energy of Reiki.

Items like watches create a closed circuit, which reduces the flow of life energy. Earrings are also a problem. The pierced ears interfere with the flow of energy. The ears are very important in many therapies such as acupuncture that utilize meridians and must be kept unencumbered.

It is recommended that you remove your shoes if they are made from leather. Even in other instances, they may be removed if it helps you feel more comfortable.

Wash Hands

Washing hands serves two purposes. Clean, washed hands are more sensitive, and will help to feel the energy flow more strongly. Dirty, sticky hands make it very difficult to sense the energy flow.

Apart from increasing sensitivity, washing hands also serves the purpose of cleansing your hands of germs and energies which you might have picked up from others. During the course of the day, one comes in touch with several people or objects which are touched by others. This affects our aura. Washing hands removes such influences.

Drink Water

Reiki Healing cleanses your body, and drinking water helps flush out the toxins from your body in the easiest manner. It is best if the healer and the patient both drink a glass of water each, before the healing.

Say the Attitude of Gratitude

Attitude of gratitude comprises three sentences.

"Thank you (*Reiki channel's name*) for being here
Thank you Reiki for being here
Thank you (*name of the person being healed; for self-healing, the Reiki channel's name is taken again*) for being here"

Thus, while you are doing self- healing, your name comes in the first and third sentence. For e.g., if your name is Meera, the attitude of gratitude will be,

"Thank you Meera for being here
Thank you Reiki for being here
Thank you Meera for being here"
Attitude of gratitude is said with the hands in Namaste position.

The Steps

Laying hands on your body with the intent to heal automatically activates Reiki flow. When you lift the hands, the flow stops. Once the flow starts, you may feel heat sensations. When the palms remain longer in the place, other sensations begin.

Different feelings of heat, cold, water flowing, static electricity, tingling, vibrations, magnetism etc., may be felt if you are sensitive enough. There are some people who may not be sensitive to these feelings. If you don't get sensations, don't think that it is because of lack of energy flow.

Once you are attuned by a qualified Reiki Teacher, the energy will definitely flow. But depending on your sensitivity, you may or may not feel the energy flow. Even if you don't feel anything, just keep doing daily practice. Within a week, either you or those around you will notice the changes in you that Reiki is bringing about.

In this respect, it is very important that you do as much Reiki healing for others as possible. Some of them will definitely be sensitive enough to feel the Reiki flow and give you the feedback. This will boost your confidence in the early stages of your practice.

The self-healing practice involves healing the seven chakra-points in the front as well as the back. The crown is not repeated.

Start with the **attitude of gratitude**.

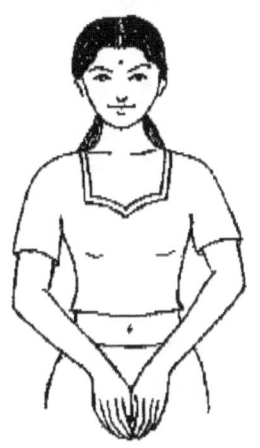

1.   A Reiki healing session begins with the palms placed over the groin for women, and at the joint between the thighs and torso for men. Slightly cup your hands and intend for the energy to flow. This radiates energy to the first chakra, the root.

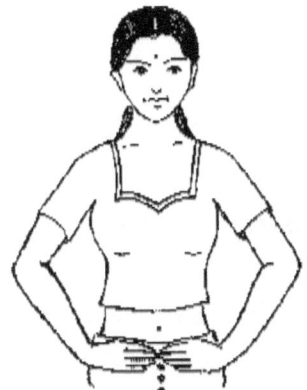

2.   The second position is over the hara chakra, which is located about three finger-widths below the navel. Move your hands one by one to this point. The middle fingers of both hands touch gently.

3.   The third position is the solar plexus, between the lower rows of ribs and about three finger-widths above the navel.

4.   The fourth position is the heart chakra, located just below the breast line with the middle fingers touching the lower end of the sternum.

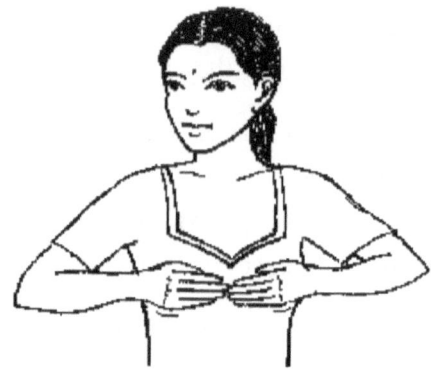

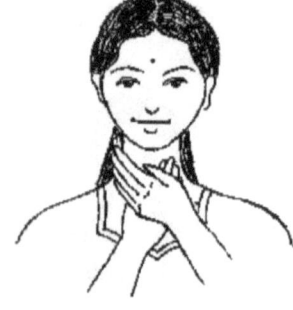

5.   The fifth position covers the throat chakra and is located at the base of the neck.

6.   In the sixth position, the palms placed over the face. This radiates energy to the third eye or brow chakra.

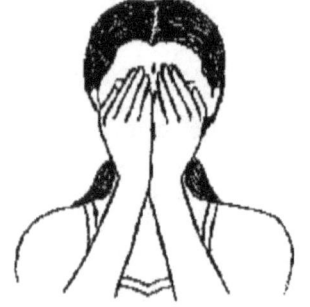

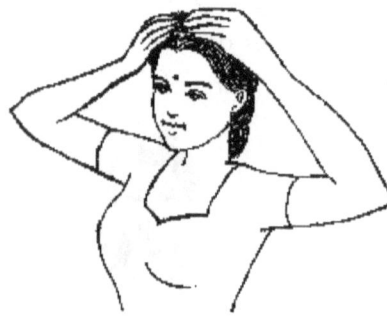

7.   The seventh position is over the temple and covers the crown chakra. Remove the palms one by one and place your palms on either side of the head, in the temple region, with the middle fingers touching each other at the front of the crown chakra.

Now that we are done with the front chakras, we begin healing the back chakras.

8.   The eighth position, the back root chakra is located at the base of the spine, so simply place your hands as far down your spine as you can, without sitting on your hands.

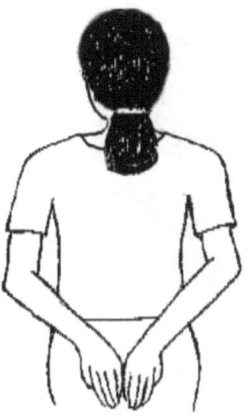

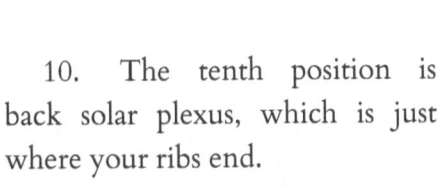

9.   The ninth position is along the belt-line on your lower back.

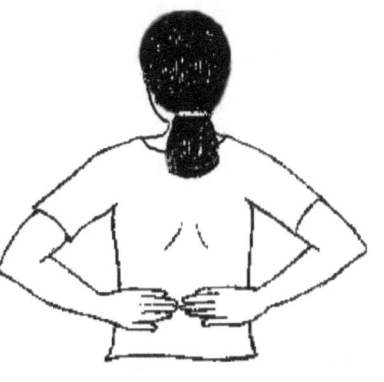

10.   The tenth position is back solar plexus, which is just where your ribs end.

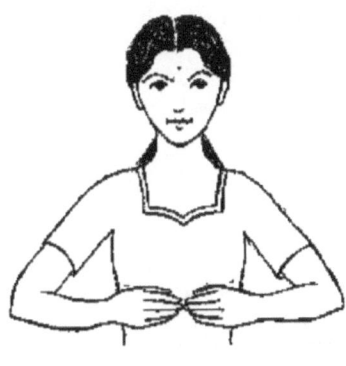

11.   The eleventh position is the back heart chakra. Since it is nearly impossible to reach this position, and definitely not comfortable even if you can, place your hands on the front heart chakra instead, bringing your complete focus to the back heart region and requesting the energy to flow there.

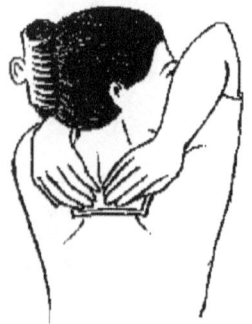

12. The twelfth position is the back of the throat chakra. It is located at the top of the shoulder blades and shoulder muscles on either side of the neck. Place your hands at the base of your neck, fingertips touching.

13. In the thirteenth twelfth position we cover the back of the head, including the occipital lobe. This radiates energy to the back of the third eye chakra. Hands may be placed such that your fingers point towards the top of your head, or such that the hands are in opposite directions, with the edge of the left little finger touching the edge of the right thumb.

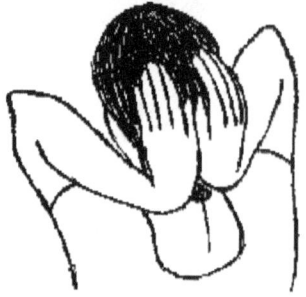

Apart from these thirteen traditional Reiki positions, knees, ankles and feet, when treated, serve to balance you after energizing the upper positions and reconnect you with mother earth.

This is the complete self-Reiki treatment and you will become familiar with the positions soon. On completion of the treatment, say the attitude of gratitude again.

'<*Your name*> is healed fully and completely. It is so.
Thank you Reiki. Thy will be done.
Thank you <*your name*> for being here.
Thank you Reiki for being here.
Thank you <*your name*> for being here.

Moving From One Point to Another

The sensations at each chakra generally last from 5 to 10 minutes on each position. Cessation of the sensation means flow of the energy needed by that particular position is complete. Then you can move the palm to the next position.

If you had not felt any sensations, follow your intuition. As long as you feel good while keeping your hands in one position or as long as you don't feel like removing your palms from there, keep them there. Also, when the energy flow is complete, you may heave a sigh. Then move the palms to the next position.

Sometimes your palms may feel glued to one position. In such a case, do not struggle, be patient. Make the move when your palms feel free. This is just an indication that the particular area needs more Reiki energy for healing.

How many days should I practice?

This is a common question asked during attunements. As I am a dentist, this question translates in my mind as, 'How many days should I brush my teeth?' If you want healthy teeth, you have to brush every day because disease causing bacteria and foodstuffs are always present in the mouth.

Similarly, disease-causing bacteria are there in our environment. We are surrounded by negative emotions like anger, jealousy, hatred etc. We fall sick when there is imbalance between the body and the environment, between the elements of the body (air, water, earth, fire and ether) or between the physical, mental, emotional and spiritual states.

A Reiki healing brings unmatched balance and harmony into our lives, thus gifting us with health, contentment and happiness.

After the attunement, twenty one days of continuous practice is necessary to attain a minimum level of channelling capacity. During this period, cleansing of the body chakras takes place. Each of the seven major chakras takes approximately three days for cleansing. For this reason, Reiki healing should be done at least once a day, if not more. Healing others as much as possible is also recommended, as it helps in the cleansing process.

The twenty-one day practice after the attunement has to be continuous. If you miss a day or two in between, you have to start again for twenty-one consecutive days. Once this initial chakra-healing phase is over, there is no harm in missing the practice once in a while. But once you start feeling the effects of Reiki, you wouldn't want to miss a single day of practice!

This millennium is marked by accelerated growth and change. Just like the water we drink and the air we breathe, Universal Life Force Energy has become a necessity in today's life style to maintain our mental balance and inner happiness. This energy has always been there for us, but we have somehow forgotten how to access it. The Usui method of natural healing is a practice that helps us regain the access so that we no longer have to suffer its lack.

But I can't find the time!

If we think carefully, this is a very poor excuse. We have time to watch soap operas on television, to read the newspaper, to gossip, and surf the Internet. But we have no time left for Reiki? Finding time for Reiki is just a matter of resetting our priorities. Once Reiki becomes a priority, we'll always find the time.

However, in case it is still too hard to spare half an hour for a daily practice, there is a way out.

We have listed 13 points for practice in this book, including the front and back chakras, and an additional 4 points, viz., ears, knees, ankles and soles. If you are hard-pressed for time, you may do self-healing for the front chakras of the body, i.e. the crown to root chakra. This makes it 7 points, and even if you give Reiki for 3 minutes per chakra, it still adds up to only 21 minutes, which is very achievable. In the worst case, you may split this into two parts, doing 4 chakras in the morning and the remaining 3 in the evening.

The next day, do the self-healing for the back chakras, repeating only the crown chakra. Again, this leaves you with 7 points to heal. If you have time left after the self-healing, you may heal the additional points listed (ears, knees, ankles, soles). On every weekend, make sure you do the complete self-healing.

If you practice Reiki at the end of the day and if you find that you are too tired to place your hands at the chakras, give Reiki to your knees for about 10 minutes. By the end of it, you will be in a position to do self-healing.

HEALING OTHERS

Both the person who is treating and the one receiving treatment should not cross their arms and legs. They should drink water before commencing treatment.

- Wash your hands
- Internally state the attitude of gratitude.
  'Thank you <*your name*> for being here.
  Thank you Reiki for being here.
  Thank you <*receiver's name*> for being here'.

For healing others, we adopt a top-down approach, starting from the crown and moving towards the feet. This is because the top-down healing brings deep relaxation and allows the person to fall asleep, which consequently opens them up to deeper healing.

The person being treated should best (most conveniently) be lying down. In case this is not possible, they can be seated sideways in a chair so that both front and back are accessible to the healer. Start the process by laying of the cupped hands in the sequence that follows.

You may choose to touch the client during healing or place our hands at a distance of about 2-3 inches away from the body. Both work just fine, but when you hold our hands at a distance, it is easier to sense the flow of energy. Sometimes family members prefer being touched as it gives them a feeling of comfort but in most other cases the client is also more relaxed when the hands are maintained at a distance.

If you prefer touching the client while healing, always seek permission before you begin.

Healing others is a simple process:

- Begin with a wish for the person to be healed.

- Wait for the feedback, or for about three to five minutes, keep the hands at each position.

- When you feel that the chakra is filled with energy, move gently onto the next, one hand at a time, always maintaining contact.

The Steps

As usual, start with the **attitude of gratitude**.

1. Slightly cup your hands and place them over the crown chakra. This picture shows the hands touching the head for ease of understanding, but many people, especially children, have a sensitive crown and it is best to place hands about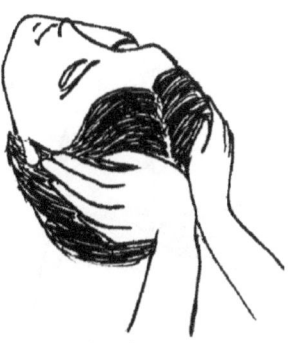

3-4 inches away from the body.

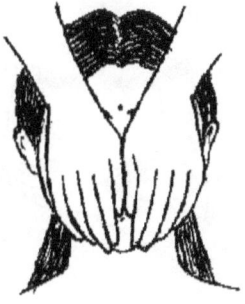

2. Next, place it over the face. Again, the direction could be as shown or if one is standing on the side of the person, the hands would be placed horizontally across the face.

3. Place your hands over the throat chakra. The direction does not matter. One could also stand on the receiver's side and place the hands similar to the next position.

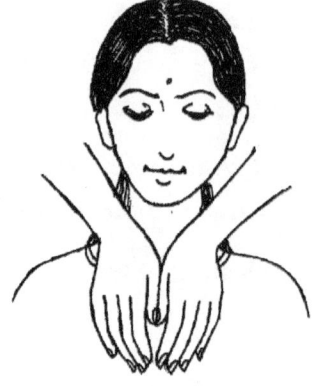

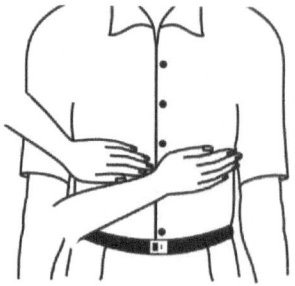

4. Move one by one to the heart chakra. Some people have a very sensitive heart and it may be wise not to place your hands too close to the body.

5. Next, move to the solar plexus. This will be at the bottom of the ribcage.

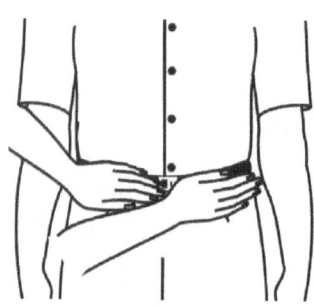

6. The hara chakra will be roughly in alignment with the belt. Move your hands to this position, one by one.

7. Next, move to the root chakra.

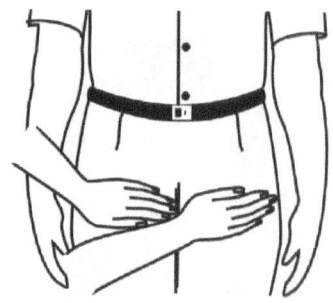

8. Spiralling

The next step is called spiralling, which balances the energies while healing. This step is not required while healing oneself.

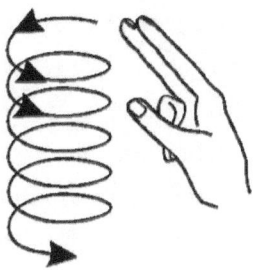

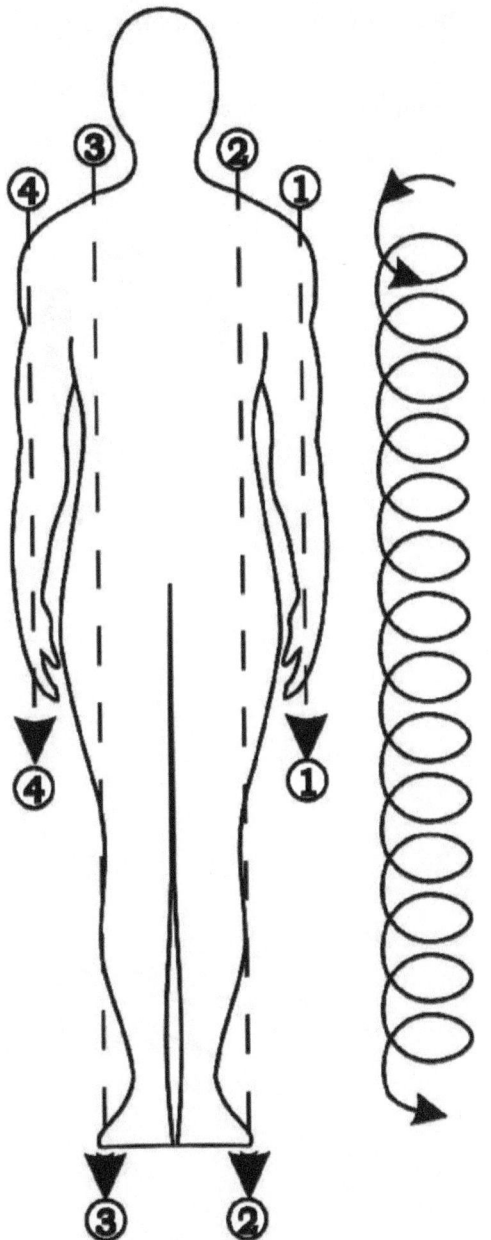

Spiraling allows free movement of the Reiki energy through the physical body of the receiver, helps the aura to expand along with the body and assists the patient to come out of the spacey feeling.

Upon completing front body Reiki, stand on the receiver's right side. Place your left palm on the receiver's right shoulder. With the first two fingers of your right hand, draw rapid anti-clockwise spirals, a few inches from the receiver's body:

1. from the receiver's left shoulder to finger tips.
2. from left shoulder to toes.
3. from right shoulder to toes.
4. from right shoulder to finger tips.

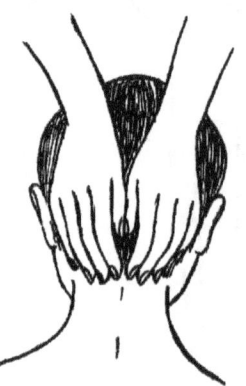

9. After spiralling, ask the client to turn over their right side (so that it is a clockwise movement) and lie on their belly. Since we have already healed the crown, we now start with the back of the brow chakra.

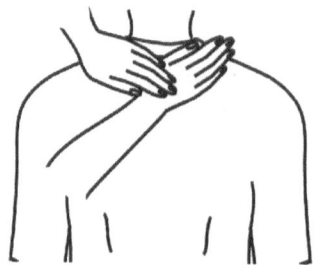

10. Start with the back throat chakra and move hands down in sequences as for the front body Reiki treatment.

11. As mentioned before, the heart chakra is sensitive. This applies to the back heart as well. If you are touching the receiver on the back heart, first ascertain that he/ she is comfortable with this. position.

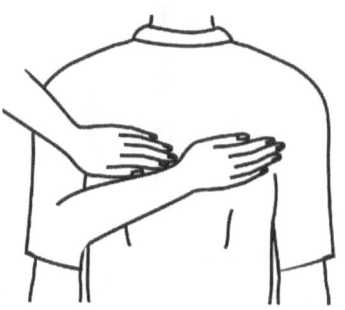

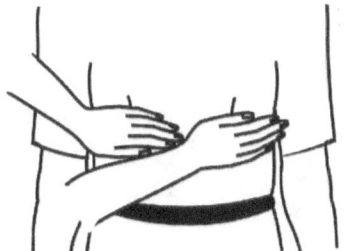

12. Next, heal the back solar chakra

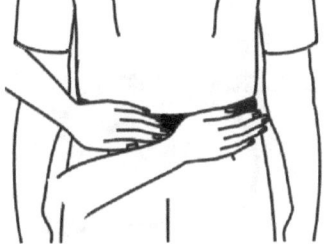

13. The back hara chakra is where the belt is usually worn.

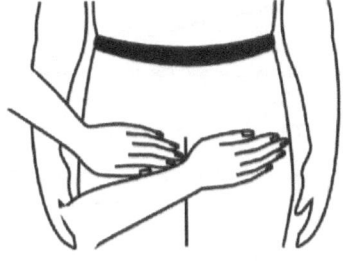

14. Finally, heal the root chakra

As an optional step, after finishing with the root chakra position, you can heal the back of knees and on the soles to ground energies of the receiver.

15. Balancing

Next, we balance the chakras. Energy is stored in the spine. It is good to relax the spine and release stored energy by balancing it.

Place your palms on the receiver's back, left palm over the third eye chakra and right palm over the root chakra. Slowly allow your palms to rise up. At some point you may feel a change in the sensation in your hands. Pause there, keeping both palms at the same level. Mentally declare, '(Receiver's name)'s third eye and root chakras are balanced. It is so.'

Now, move the left palm over to throat chakra and the right palm to the hara chakra. Mentally declare, '(Receiver's name)'s throat and hara chakras are balanced. It is so'.

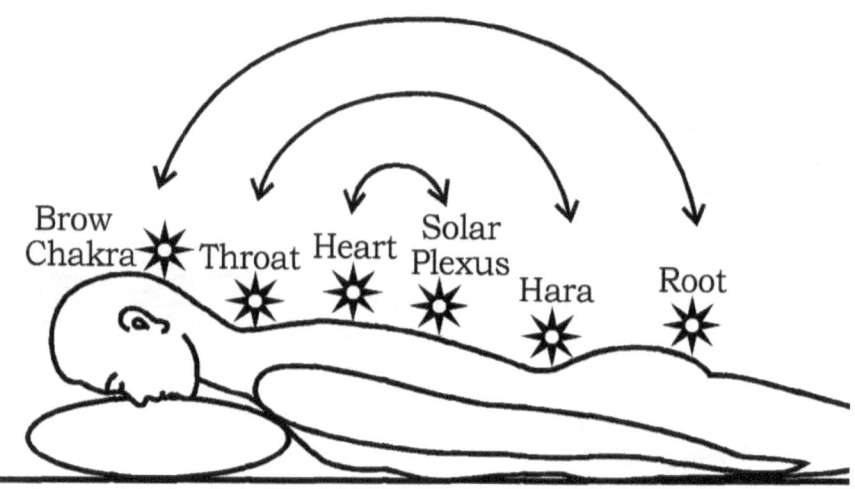

Move the left palm over to the heart chakra and the right palm to the solar plexus chakra. Mentally declare,'(Receiver's name)'s heart and solar plexus chakras are balanced. It is so.'

Place your right palm lightly on receiver's heart chakra area on his back, then place your left palm on top of your right palm.

Mentally declare '(Receiver's name)'s chakras are balanced; he is healed fully and completely. It is so. Thank you Reiki. Thy will be done.'

Place your left hand over the receiver's left shoulder. Hold the first two fingers of the right hand in a V-shape and with them; draw three vertical lines from the back throat chakra to the back root chakra.

If the receiver has diabetes and is on insulin, draw the lines from the back root chakra towards the back throat chakra, as this movement often causes a sudden sugar drop and a person on insulin might feel uneasy.

After completing chakra balancing, place your right hand lightly on the hara chakra of the receiver. This is to store any extra energies in the hara.

16. End with the attitude of gratitude and wash your hands.

17. If the receiver is asleep at the end of the session, leave him/her undisturbed for as long as possible.

19. Both the Reiki channel and the receiver should drink a glass of water after the Reiki treatment.

Reiki to food, plants, animals & infants

Many people venture into Reiki for getting relief from physical ailments. This relief is brought about by balancing effects of the Universal Life Force Energy. If we take a deeper look, this energy is nothing but vibration. And vibration, as we know, is present in every matter, whether living or non-living. All matter is vibration at different levels of density. Hence Reiki can penetrate anything.

Reiki can have an effect on plants, animals and food. It is up to your imagination and use of your intuition to explore the limitless applications of Reiki.

If you give Reiki to seeds by holding them between the palms of your hands before planting, they tend to grow into healthier plants. Seed sprouts and plants can be treated by holding your hands above them. Cut flowers will last longer with Reiki.

If animals are given Reiki, generally they become very calm and relaxed. Reiki can be used to clear the environment around the patient in a hospital to remove any negative energy.

Rechargeable cells can be energized by Reiki. Hold your hands above your plate of food before you eat and you will enhance the food with the Universal Life Force Energy. Give Reiki to your restless toddler and see its calming effect.

BODY, EMOTIONS, DISEASES

Long before the physical manifestation of any disease, it starts in the emotions/attitudes of the person. It is therefore, useful to know the relationship of accumulated emotions and the diseases that manifest. While healing someone through Reiki, always allow your feedback to guide you. You may give more Reiki energy to the associated chakras in case of a lack of sensations.

When there is no apparent cause for disease in terms of attitudinal or emotional pattern, or where it is very mildly present, the disease must be understood as deeply karmic in nature, requiring persistent healing.

Remember that Reiki channels are not doctors. Never discourage the client from continuing his on-going therapies, especially in severe or difficult conditions. Just add Reiki healing to the other measures taken. Do not give judgmental diagnosis to clients.

An ailment will reflect the individual's inner emotional condition, inner distress, and inner attitudes that need to be healed. Even accidents are sharply delivered results of our inner condition. Accidents are brought about by ourselves to help us question our present course. When you find the inner reason for the accident, analyse the problem and work on resolving it. It may be due to inability to speak up for one's self, rebellion of authority or belief in violence.

When a particular organ is affected, the feeling or aspect associated with that organ is already traumatized, before the physical involvement takes place. The prior subtle emotional background always appears first. If this is corrected and healed, then the physical involvement can be averted. In this manner, Reiki healing has great preventive value.

Body parts & Associated Emotions

When trying to understand the ailments, it is useful to remember that:

1. The body part affected is directly related to an emotional state of the individual and his life condition.

2. The right side of the body is associated with the masculine side of the personality. Problems with this side usually deal with situations under one's control, the individual's own self, family, personal goals, objectives etc.,

3. The left side of the body is associated with the feminine side of the personality. Problems with this side of the body are due to situations out of one's control, and usually have to do with the rest of the world- the 'others'.

Following are the emotions/ issues related to parts of the body.

Face: Expression of our personality and how we face the world

Forehead (third eye, occipital lobes, temples): Mental, intellectual expression, nervous system, will power, wisdom, intuition and mystic powers.

Eyes: How we view the world, and what we see around us

Nose: Related to heart. Sense of smell, sexual response, self-recognition

Mouth: Survival issues, capacity to take in new ideas and concepts

Jaws: Emotional and verbal communication; Fear of expressing oneself; Survival issues

Neck: The mental and the emotional come together. Withheld feelings give stiffness here

Ears: Balance in life. Capacity to hear and accept the heard

Arms and hands: Extensions of heart centre, expression of love, emotion, giving and receiving, creativity.

Shoulders: Responsibility area; relationships

Upper back: (Thymus) Storehouse of unconscious emotions and tensions. Anger.

Lower back: Storehouse of unresolved emotions. Relationship issues.

Base of spine/ root chakra: Essential bodily survival issues. Seat of kundalini energy; Destiny, seed karma

Chest: Relationship issues; Power centre for women

Lung: The ability to take in life, fear of taking in life.

Heart: Love; Seat of the soul, spiritual being

Solar plexus: Power and control issues, practical wisdom. Immediately experienced emotions of fear, hatred, anger, jealousy, envy, courage, perseverance etc.,

Abdomen/Hara: Seat of deepest emotions, hurt feelings; Power centre for men;

Liver: Seat of anger, chronic complaining; Fault finding to deceive yourself; Digestion and transmutation of lower emotions to higher; Emotional indigestion at all levels.

Spleen and Pancreas: Anger, helplessness.

Genitals: Survival and root chakra issues; Fear of life/ existence.

Thighs: Personal strength and trust in one's own abilities. Self-confidence

Knees: Fear of death. Fear of death of one's own ego or own self / consciousness; fear of change, moving ahead; Knees represent pride and ego. Inability to bend; Personal responsibility issues

Calves: Addictions/ attachments; Fear of change, moving ahead.

Lower leg: Fear of action; Capacity for moving towards goals

Ankles: Balance, discrimination in life's activities

Feet: Connecting with and reaching one's goals; Fear of completion of activities; Procrastination, laziness

Problems & associated emotions

Accidents: Inability to speak up for one's self; rebellion of authority; belief in violence

Everything happens to us for a reason, including accidents. These are brought about by ourselves to help us question our present course. When you find the inner reason for the accident, analyse the problem and work on resolving it. You will gain great insights and help propel yourself along your spiritual path.

Aches: Longing to be held; longing for love

Acne: Not accepting or disliking self

Addictions: Running away from self, not facing one's fears. Not knowing how to love oneself.

Aging problems: Social beliefs. Old thinking; fear of being one's self; rejection of the 'now'

AIDS: Feeling defenceless and hopeless. Denial of the true inner being, or sexual guilt

Alcoholism / abuse: Futility, guilt, inadequacy, self-rejection

Allergy & hay fever: You are allergic to someone who denies your power.

An allergy is a reaction by the body to something, which is recognized as an invader. Fighting a self-created enemy is an act of aggression, an unconscious fight against an area of life we are afraid of and do not want. Resistance is the opposite of love; love means accepting and becoming one. The substance that triggers an allergic reason is a symbol of the area of life you are avoiding and unconsciously fighting.

Look at the areas of your life which are in conflict. You will come to realize that nothing is good or bad unless you make it that way.

Alzheimer's: Refusal to deal with the world as it is.

Angina, Ischemia: Functional shortage/ lack of loving energy at back heart chakra.

Ankle problems: Inflexibility and guilt; inability to receive pleasure; lack of discrimination/ balance in activities

Anorexia: Denying the self and life. Extreme fear of rejection.

Anxiety / nervousness: Distrust in the natural flow of life.

Arteriosclerosis: Hardened narrow-mindedness.

Arm problems: Action. Right hand usually indicates regret, and left hand, helplessness.

Arthritis: Feeling unloved, criticism, resentment

Asthma: Inability to breathe for one's self. Feeling stifled. Suppressed crying.

Back (upper): Lack of emotional support, or feeling unloved. Results of stored anger, frustration and helplessness

Back (middle): Guilt. A feeling of 'get off my back'.

Back (lower): Financial woes and concerns.

Baldness: Fear, tension. Trying to control everything and not trusting in the process of life.

Blackheads (pimples): Small outbursts of anger.

Blood problems: Lack of joy; lack of ideas

Blood pressure: High (hypertension): Longstanding emotional problems not solved. Blood pressure is the pressure of the blood against the inner walls of the blood vessels, especially of the arteries during different phases of contraction of the heart.

High blood pressure arises when you haven't expressed your thoughts and emotions over a long period of time. You are constantly living on the brink of conflict, without coming to any kind of conclusion, under constant pressure.

Blood pressure: Low: Lack of love as a child. Defeatism. "What's the use? It won't work anyway."

Low blood pressure is caused by trying to avoid facing problems. It occurs when you have a lack of vital energy, stamina and cannot assert yourself. It can also indicate an attempt to avoid sexuality. It signifies defeatism – thinking, "what is the use? It won't work anyway".

Bone breaks: Rebelling against authority.

Bowel problems: Fear of letting go

Breast (left): Feeling unloved, refusal to nourish oneself. Putting everyone else first.

Breast (right): Over protection, over bearing, difficulty in giving love.

Breast tumour: Blockage or trauma to woman's purpose of life, of the outflow of loving energy.

Breathing problems: Fear or the refusal to take in life; not feeling worthy to take up space

Bronchitis: Inflamed family environment.

Bruises: Self-punishment.

Bulimia: Hopeless terror. Purging self-hatred.

This is caused by a hunger for life, love and emotional nourishment. There is a feeling of emptiness inside which you desperately try to fill. You may be insecure and afraid of loss.

Learn to accept and love yourself as you are; you'll find it easier to open the limitations of your ego and take in spiritual nourishment. Know that there is an inexhaustible source of love and fulfilment, and it's inside you.

Burns: Anger, burning up inside.

Calculi in salivary glands: New ideas, concepts hard to digest, but individual does not openly challenge them.

Cancer: Deep hurt, secret or grief; long-standing resentment. Carrying hatreds. Thinking, "what is the use?" Anger, self-consumption; a desire to destroy the life force by totally turning away from the "I am" (god-self); absence of self-love.

The cosmic fire does not feed the root chakra and is distinctly disrupted by the emotions of remorse, fear and internalised anger stemming from deep-rooted and long-term issues of the ego, yet unresolved by forgiveness.

To not deal with these issues, holds the pattern for the energy to destroy life force. True forgiveness is complete and healing will result.

Carpal tunnel: Anger at life's seeming injustices.

Cataracts: Does not like what he sees in the world.

Cavities in teeth: New ideas/ concepts are hard to take in, become survival issues openly if old concepts and belief systems are threatened

Cervical abnormalities: Poorly defined boundaries in relationships, relationships and activities that detract from well-being, guilt about sexual pleasure

Cervical ribs, shoulder pains: Carrying assumed burdens and responsibilities, not rightfully one's own; relationship problems

Cervical spondylosis: Inability to express what one feels due to conflict between the intellect and heart. (cervical 5, 6, 7 vertebrae corresponding to throat chakra)

Cholesterol (high): Clogging the channels of joy.

Chronic diseases: A refusal to change; fear of the future; not feeling safe

Circulation: Lack of joy or the lack of circulation of ideas.

Colds: Too much going on at once. Confusion and disorder.

Colic: Mental irritation. Annoyance with surroundings

Colour blindness: Lack of discrimination/ balance; Reiki the ankles, particularly effective for colour-blind people

Coma: Fear. Trying to escape from something or someone

Cold sores: Festering angry words, fear of expressing them.

Common colds & flu: Cleansing and release

A stagnant conflict is loosening up. Look at colds and the flu as a cleansing of your body. Your body is purging the toxic chemicals from drugs, food, air, water, cigarettes, alcohol that you continually ingest.

Bless this time of purification, as it will allow you to be in continuing good health. Let the body rest; healing will be faster.

Constipation: Refusing to release old ideas

This often has to do with greediness, stinginess, wanting to hold on to things (usually material possessions). You may also have difficulty letting go of old ideas and may repress problems, fearing the outcome if they were to surface. You must learn to let go.

Allow life to flow through you and you will find the security and riches you are seeking, within yourself. Your true sustenance comes from God (source of life, love, oneness) and not from outside sources (money, relationships, status).

Coronary artery disease: Blockage in the flow of love- inability to receive or accept love.

Cough: A desire to bark at the world. "listen to me!"

Cramps, rigidity, stiffness of calves: Does not like or adjust to natural changes taking place in life (and body) - as in pregnancy

Resistance to moving forward to new condition/ state in life; attachment to the old; self- control issues as in habits, addictions, temper etc., and over-control

Death and the dying process: One of our most important life processes is that of dying (transformation of consciousness). Your physical living body is in a continual process of cycles of birthing and dying (cells, hair). Your emotional body is in various stages of birthing and dying emotions. So, too, are your thoughts (mental) as well as each level of your being, according to its nature.

Degenerative retinopathy, retinal haemorrhage: Does not like what is seen in his personal life; does not like his view of himself

Depression: Anger you don't feel you have a right to have. Hopelessness. Lack of ability to work because of lack of self-confidence. Heal solar plexus, back heart and hara.

Diabetes: Longing for what might have been. No sweetness left in life.

This indicates a wish for love, paired with the inability to let oneself be loved. Those who do not love, turn sour.

Don't wait for love to come from outside; let love in and all around you. Let go of the past and accept that fun, love and affection are fundamental basics of life.

Diarrhoea: Fear and rejecting. Running off or away from something/someone

Digestive disorders: Inability to digest events. Suppressed anger. Vomiting is usually a purging of suppressed or unexpressed emotions. The solar plexus is involved for all digestive disorders, mental-emotional- physical and all acute problems including fever and infections.

Dizziness: Flighty, scattered thinking.

Drug addictions: Lack of grounding and self-love. Result in closing down of back heart chakra and root chakra.

Ear problems: Not wanting to hear. Anger or too much turmoil

Elbow problems: Not being flexible, not able to change directions or accept new experiences.

Eye (astigmatism): Fear of "seeing" the self

Eye (cataracts): Inability to see ahead with joy

Eye problems: (children) not wanting to see what's going on in the family

Eye (farsighted): Fear of the present

Eye (near-sighted): Fear of the future.

Eye sty: Looking at life through angry eyes. Angry at someone.

Fainting: Fear, can't cope, blacking out what's really going on.

Fat: Over sensitivity. Often represents fear and shows a need for protection; fear may be a cover for hidden anger and resistance to forgive

Fatigue (chronic fatigue syndrome): This can be caused by a possible closing down of the throat chakra level, creating an energy block. You may experience a total lack of motivation overshadowed with justifications of probable failure.

Emotional stimulation with an objective and goal is needed. Usually caused by dissatisfaction with and dwelling on circumstances and situations in the present (or past) and projecting the hopelessness into the future.

Feet problems: Fear of the future or not wanting to move forward towards goals, while life events overwhelmingly indicate movement is essential.

Female problems: Denial of the self and rejecting the feminine aspects within.

Fevers & infections: Anger, burning up.

Fibroids: Nursing a hurt from a partner, a blow to the feminine ego

Finger (thumb): Worry, always thinking. Being 'under someone's thumb'.

Finger (index): Fear of authority, or egotistical; abusing your authority.

Flu: Responding to mass negativity. Putting too much faith in statistics.

Gall stones/ pancreatitis: Undigested emotion; deep unforgiven hurt solidifies as gallstones: + anger = pancreatitis.

Gas pain (flatulence): Undigested ideas or concerns.

Gastritis: Prolonged uncertainty; a feeling of doom

Glaucoma: Inability to weep, unshed tears

Gray hair: Stress, feeling under pressure and strain.

Growths: Nursing old hurts; building resentments.

Growth disorders and basic health disorders come from root chakra. (skeletal system, circulatory system, bodily form and development)

Gum problems: Inability to back up decisions. Being wishy-washy about life.

Hand problems: Grasping on to tight, not wanting to let go. Not 'handling' things well.

Headaches: Self-criticism. Not wanting to accept what is going on

Heart attack: Squeezing all the joy out of life, in favour of money or position.

Inability to receive/ accept love has reached a severely settled traumatic stage; squeezing all the joy out of the heart in favour of money and position; lack of joy; belief in strain and stress.

In such a condition, giving reiki by placing the right hand on the back heart chakra and the left hand on the solar plexus chakra, can be a life-saving procedure and facilitates extremely good recovery.

Heartburn (reflux): Clutching onto fear. Not trusting in the process of life.

Heart problems: Lack of joy, dealing with issues from anger, not love. Indicate heartlessness, hard-heartedness and doing things half-hearted. These characteristics are the result of protracted emotional life and a fight for survival. Ask yourself if your head, heart, intellect and emotions are in balance. Do you live with all your heart? Are you able to question your heart freely or do you need to become ill first?

Haemorrhoids: Fear of deadlines. Afraid to let go and move on.

Hernia: Ruptured relationships, strain, burdens, incorrect creative expression

Hip problems: Fear of going forward in major decisions.

Hyperactivity: Feeling pressured and frantic

Hyperventilation: Resisting change. Not being able to take it all in.

Impotence: Sexual guilt or pressure, feeling spite against a previous mate; purpose of life is deeply traumatized. Heal hara, kidneys.

Indigestion: Dread or anxiety about a recent or coming event

Infection: Irritation, anger or annoyance about a recent situation.

Infertility/miscarriage: Insufficient energy, ambivalence about impact of pregnancy on lifestyle and body image, hanging on to grief or loss

Influenza: Response to mass negativity and beliefs; fear.

Insomnia: Coming from over-active thinking, mental activity (which is subtle speech). Fear, guilt. Not trusting the process of life.

Joints: Unable to change and be flexible in direction of life.

Kidney disorders: Relationship problems and issues not dealt with/ painful to deal with openly.

Kidney stones: Lumps of unresolved anger.

Knee problems: Inability to bend, stubborn pride

Laryngitis: Fear of speaking up.

Left side of body: The feminine side. Represents receptivity, taking in, women, mother, love.

Leg problems: Fear of the future, not being able to carry things forward.

Leukaemia: Brutally killing inspiration. "What's the use?"

Liver problems: (hepatitis) resistance to change. Fear, anger, hatred. Liver is the seat of anger and rage.

Lung problems: Depression, grief or fear of life. Not feeling worthy.

Lymphatic problems: A warning that the mind needs to be re-centred on the essentials of life. Life and joy.

Menopause: Fear of no longer being wanted.

Mental alertness & senility: Returning to the "safety" of childhood. Demanding care and attention.

Migraine headache: Sexual fears, or fear of being close, letting someone in too close. Feeling driven or pressured. Emotional indigestion; resisting the flow of life, dislike of being driven, sexual fears; heal the liver under such circumstances.

Menstrual imbalance/PMS: Rejection of one's femininity. Guilt or feeling "dirty".

Nausea: Fear, rejecting an idea or experience.

Neck problems: Refusing to see another's side or position. Stubbornness. Who/what is being a pain in the neck?

Osteoporosis: Feeling there is no support left in life.

Overweight problems: Fear, feeling a deep need for emotional protection; running away from feelings, insecurity

Pain: Self-punishment, feeling emotional guilt.

Paralysis: Extreme hopelessness and helplessness. Heal back heart chakra, thymus front and back, and root chakra.

Pimples: Dislike/ disgust at one's body/ bodily parts, processes or changes taking place in the body, as in puberty- (liver + hara).

Post nasal drip: Inner crying; belief in being a victim

Prostate enlargement: Mental fears weakening the masculinity. Sexual pressure and feelings of guilt or inadequacy.

Rashes, urticaria: Inability to digest emotions- all arising from the liver (and solar plexus).

Respiratory illnesses: Fear of taking in life fully; depression, grief, not feeling worthy of taking in life

Sagging lines: (on the face) sagging thoughts in the mind; resentment of life

Sciatica: Being hypocritical; fear of money and the future.

Seizures: Running away from the self, family or from life.

Shoulder problems: Carrying the weight of the world on your shoulders. Feeling like life is a burden.

Sinus problems/ deviated septum: Irritation with someone, usually someone close to you; unsure of personal identity; unsure as to what options should be taken professionally, career-wise or occupationally

Slipped spinal disk, lumbar spondylosis: 'purpose of life' traumatized, refusal to acknowledge unresolved emotions and related issues

Skin conditions: Anxiety, fear, feeling threatened.

Slipped disk: Feeling unsupported in life.

Sore throat: Holding in angry words. Feeling unable to express the self.

Smoking: The lungs symbolize the idea of freedom and communication which you are trying to conjure up by smoking, but your wishes become more and more nebulous in the process.

Become aware of what you want, and then you can create it in your life. Genuine communication can only take place in an atmosphere of clarity.

Snoring: Stubborn refusal to let go of old patterns.

Stomach & intestinal problems: Dread, fear of the new, or not feeling nourished.

Stroke: Insecurity, lack of self-expression. Not being allowed to cry.

Suicidal tendency: Small or weak root chakra

Teeth problems: Being indecisive, not being able to break down ideas for analysis and decisions.

Testicular problems: Not accepting masculine principles, or the masculinity within.

Thyroid problems: Humiliation. Feeling repressed or put down. Feeling as if you never get to do what you want.

Trigeminal neuralgia: Inability to face the world due to damage of our self-image, self-worth. Energize heart and hara chakras to draw up and heal the emotion and thinking. Place your right hand on heart chakra and left hand on hara chakra

Tumours: Nursing old hurts and shocks. Building on remorse

Ulcers: Fear, a strong belief that you are not good enough. Anxious to please. A strong belief that you are not good enough. What is eating away at you? Emotionally being eaten away by holding in anger and unpleasant thought-forms.

You need to come to the understanding of where the stress is that is disrupting your harmony, and release it via some creative outlet.

Urinary problems: Feeling pissed off! Usually at the opposite sex or lover.

Uterine, ovarian disorders, prostrate disorders: Self-blame, guilt ('can't live with myself'); trauma to the individual's purpose of life; unfulfilled/ traumatized purposes and desires

Varicose veins: Standing in a situation you hate. Feeling over worked and overburdened.

Vertigo: Ears and third eye are secondary areas after ankles (primary area) if vertigo is caused by mental- emotional trauma due to hearing unpleasant things. Lack of discrimination/balance (third eye, temples)

Warts: Little expressions of hate.

Wounds: Anger and guilt at self

POINTS TO REMEMBER

Drink as much water as possible

Drinking a lot of water is important during Reiki treatment, for the Reiki channel as well as the receiver. Apart from the other benefits, it helps flush out toxins from the body, and hence eases the cleansing process.

Keep your hands and legs uncrossed

Hands and legs should not be crossed as it can hinder free flow of Reiki energy. Yoga poses like the lotus pose (*padmasana*) or easy pose (sukhasana) are however, alright.

After the Attunement

When you are attuned, if you are sensitive to the energy flow, for a few days or for twenty-one days, you will be acutely aware of the Reiki flow. Then you may feel as if the energy is not flowing or it is very mild.

When you are attuned, there is a sudden surge of energy flow and the chakra cleansing takes place for twenty- one days. After you reach a certain energy level, if you practice Reiki daily, you don't need too much of daily cleansing. Then the mild energy flow may not be sufficient to make you feel its presence.

Reiki heals and balances

Reiki energy can never be used to harm somebody. It is purely positive energy and cannot be used for negative purposes. Also, there is no such thing as 'right' or 'wrong' reiki. There are several variations in Reiki, and all of them are positive. You learn the stream that is best for your progress.

There is no such thing as 'too much Reiki'

The body will take up only as much energy as it needs at a particular point of time. You need not have doubts that too much of Reiki can cause some problem.

Never take the credit for healing anybody

As Reiki channels, we are just transmitting the energy to the needy person. All the changes that subsequently happen are because of the Reiki, and not because of you.

Similarly, if you don't see the expected results immediately, don't blame yourself, and don't harbour any doubts that 'your' Reiki is not working. In such cases, Reiki is usually healing the root of the problem, which is often hidden and hence related changes are hard to notice. Give it time.

Keep your expectations in check

On giving Reiki, you may expect a particular result. But Reiki will go to the root cause and correct that first. When you don't see the expected result, you may think that Reiki is not working.

For example, when you give Reiki for shoulder pain, if the cause for that pain is emotional, first that person's emotional relationships will improve and later, the pain will gradually disappear. Though the person may complain that there is no immediate improvement in the shoulder pain, his close acquaintances will notice the change in his behaviour, as he will be at peace with himself.

You can practice on all days

Normally women are advised to avoid religious practices during their menstrual cycle. Practicing Reiki, however, is very helpful as it balances the energies and prevents PMS.

Practice Regularly

During the first 21 days, you must practice as much Reiki as possible so that you can maximise the cleansing benefits of Reiki.

However, this does not mean that you may now stop practicing daily once the 21 days are over. Just like a vehicle must be run every day to keep the functioning smooth, you must practice Reiki self-healing every day to maintain and increase the energy flow through your body.

If it is hard to find time to do the complete self-healing, you may practice Reiki by giving Reiki to only the front chakras of the body one day, and the back chakras the next day. This reduces the practice time to about 15-20 minutes, something very achievable in the busiest of schedules.

WHAT PEOPLE SAY

Ms Minal

I had suffered from chronic sinusitis for years. From Allopathy to Ayurveda and homeopathy, I had tried everything for a cure but the sinus problem refused to let go.

About three years back I had a major attack of sinusitis and life was unbearable because I couldn't do any work. To add to my problems, my father was hospitalised.

Beena didi, my friend (author of this book) knew about this problem. One day she gave me a call and asked me how my sinusitis was. Strangely, I realised my nose and head were clear. I felt very light and I could breathe easily. This magical change was brought about by her distant Reiki treatment. From that date till today, I have not had another attack of sinusitis.

I am a strong proponent of Reiki. I feel that Reiki can be applied to every facet of your life. Try it and enjoy the kick you get out of Reiki.

Anuradha

There was a lot of discord and misunderstanding between my in-laws and me. They would get into my way too often and attempts to resolve this by means of discussion had not helped at all. Once I started practicing Reiki on a regular basis, they began to keep to themselves and left me un-hassled. What could not be achieved by any other means was achieved through Reiki. That too without any effort in that direction!

I was a very hyper-active person until I learned Reiki, and I just could not sit down calmly without any work to do. I needed to be doing something all the time. However, after learning Reiki I find myself a lot more peaceful and can even meditate. My family is also very pleased with the change.

Priya Raju

Life brought me some uncomfortable situations at an early age. I was totally clueless, depressed, believed life was unfair to me, had many questions in my mind and heart, was afraid to stand all alone and was always seeking approval from peers. I suffered from severe back and shoulder pain.

Reiki opened up new doors in my life. I could heal myself and my past. I learned to be compassionate, respectful and loving towards myself. I learned to let go of my emotions freely and gained a lot of self-confidence.

The biggest lesson was that I learned to accept myself when I am depressed, tired and full of tears, sad and feeling low. Reiki helped me gain emotional strength, and made me capable of moving on irrespective of hardships. Reiki has helped me heal my parents, friends, a year old baby, plants and it's an amazing feeling.

Reiki has allowed light in my life. My relationship with my mother has transformed to a level where we both can put across our opinions at least and still be at peace with each other. Just taking out few minutes every day, one can not only make difference in one's own life but also contribute peace, love and light on Earth.

Arun Ananthakrishnan

Three years ago, I decided to learn Reiki with Ashwita. I had no agenda or expectations to begin with; little did I know that my life was about to change! Reiki has since had a profound impact in every aspect of my life and it would be hard to measure and quantify the extent to which the impact has been.

Life has transformed, and I have found that no matter what obstacles life throws at me, I am able to still smile and deal with it effectively.

The healing powers of Reiki certainly extend far beyond one's imagination and I truly believe in this. I believe that the healing powers of Reiki is just what each one needs to keep moving on in the right direction with a sense of well-being, health and happiness.

Nityanand Mukherjee

Four years ago, a discussion with my sister about her experiences with Reiki got me interested. Although I didn't experience any sensations, I decided to try it for 21 days. At the end of those 21 days, I was able to heal my little daughter of fever and cough, which was just the encouragement I needed.

Since then I have given Reiki healing to many people and they have been pleasantly surprised by the results! They have called it a miracle.

The most recent occasion was when I gave Reiki to a person suffering from last stage cancer. He experienced tremendous relief; his sleep improved and he was in less pain. We could not save him, but I am certain that Reiki was able to reduce his pain and suffering during his last few days.

I have several such amazing examples of things that have no explanation other than being a miracle of Reiki. Today, I'm still practical about everything and I just believe that Reiki is as practical as everything else! This energy is available, and for anything positive, Reiki works like a charm!

BIBLIOGRAPHY

1. Bodo J Baginski, Shalila Sharamon: Reiki Universal Life Energy. Mendocino, CA, Life Rhythm Publishing, 1988.
2. Diane Stein: Essential Reiki: A complete guide to an ancient healing art. CA, The Crossing Press, 1995.
3. Frank Arjava Petter: Reiki Fire. Delhi, Motilal Banarasidas Publishers, 1998
4. Martin Nazareth: Reiki. Mumbai, Perfect Health Care, 1997
5. Nalin Nirula, Renoo Nirula: The joy of Reiki. New Delhi, Full Circle, 1996
6. Nalin Nirula, Renoo Nirula: The Living Handbook of Reiki. New Delhi, The Whole Earth Company, 1998
7. Paula Horan: Empowerment through Reiki. Delhi, Motilal Banarasidas Publishers Pvt. Ltd., 1997.
8. Paula Horan: Reiki 108 Questions and Answers. Delhi, Full Circle, 1998
9. Holistic Online
    http://holistic-online.com/herb_home.htm
10. Reiki Relief (Self Healing Remedies)
    http://www.meanwell.com.au/articles/page5.html
11. Reiki Healing Energy and Illness
    http://reikithehealingpath.com/illness_causes.htm
12. Spiritual Meaning Underlying Diseases
    http://www.squidoo.com/spiritualmeaning

www.ingramcontent.com/pod-product-compliance
Lightning Source LLC
Chambersburg PA
CBHW050501290526
45786CB00006B/2392